Epilepsy

100 Elementary Principles

To Candace

Volume 12 in the Series
Major Problems in Neurology
SIR JOHN N. WALTON, T.D., M.D., D.Sc., F.R.C.P.
Consulting Editor

OTHER MONOGRAPHS IN THE SERIES

Barnett, Foster and Hudgson: **Syringomyelia,** *1973*

Dubowitz and Brooke: **Muscle Biopsy: A Modern Approach,** *1973*

Pallis and Lewis: **The Neurology of Gastrointestinal Disease,** *1974*

Hutchinson and Acheson: **Strokes,** *1975*

Gubbay: **The Clumsy Child,** *1975*

Hankinson and Banna: **Pituitary and Parapituitary Tumours,** *1976*

Donaldson: **Neurology of Pregnancy,** *1978*

Behan and Currie: **Neuroimmunology,** *1978*

Harper: **Myotonic Dystrophy,** *1979*

Cartlidge and Shaw: **Head Injury,** *1981*

Lisak and Barchi : **Myasthenia Gravis,** *1982*

Epilepsy

100 Elementary Principles

ROGER J. PORTER M.D.

Chief, Medical Neurology Branch
and
Chief, Clinical Epilepsy Section
National Institute of Neurological and
Communicative Disorders and Stroke
National Institutes of Health

W. B. Saunders Company   London Philadelphia Toronto
Mexico City Rio de Janeiro Sydney Tokyo Hong Kong

W.B. Saunders Company   33 The Avenue
Eastbourne, East Sussex BN21 3UN, England

West Washington Square
Philadelphia, PA 19105, U.S.A.

1 Goldthorne Avenue
Toronto, Ontario M8Z 5T9, Canada

Apartado 26370 — Cedro 512
Mexico 4, D.F., Mexico

Rua Evaristo da Veiga, 55–20° andar
Rio de Janeiro — RJ, Brazil

9 Waltham Street
Artarmon, N.S.W. 2064, Australia

Ichibancho Central Building, 22-1 Ichibancho
Chiyoda-ku, Tokyo 102, Japan

Second Floor Unit 2, East Asia Commercial Centre
36–60 Texaco Road, Tsuen Wan N.T., Hong Kong

First published 1984
Reprinted 1985, 1987

Typeset by First Page Ltd, Watford
Printed and bound in Great Britain by
Biddles Ltd, Guildford and King's Lynn

British Library Cataloguing in Publication Data
Porter, Roger J.
  Epilepsy.—(Major problems in neurology; 12)
  1. Epilepsy
  I. Title   II. Series
  6168′53   RC372

ISBN 0-7216-1273-3

Contents

Series Editor's Foreword

This book by Dr. Roger Porter is a monograph with a difference, and I have found it fascinating. Most of the previous volumes to have been published in this series have dealt either with individual diseases or disease processes, or with diagnostic methods, and all have been prepared in relatively standard format. When Dr. Porter originally approached me and explained his ideas relating to this book, I confess that I had some reservations about the format which he proposed to use, but these have been totally allayed by the content of the volume, which I warmly commend to a wide medical audience. Epilepsy is, after all, one the commonest disorders of the central nervous system with which not only neurologists and pediatric neurologists but also other medical specialists must frequently deal. Indeed, all primary care physicians, family doctors or general practitioners, however they are styled, as well as pediatricians, physicians in internal medicine, and also psychiatrists need to have an understanding of certain fundamental principles relating to the diagnosis and management of this condition which so commonly confronts them in their everyday clinical practice. All of these and indeed a great many other health care professionals, and, dare I say it, patients, could find much invaluable information within this book, presented in a unique, meaningful and yet readable way.

This volume cannot claim to be a textbook of epilepsy. It is, as its name implies, a comprehensive and detailed commentary upon 100 guiding principles that are of fundamental importance in the diagnosis and management of this common disorder. The presentation is detailed and explicit yet succinct and precise. The advice given is clearly expressed, and in the various sections where specific principles are outlined, the author deploys the fruits of his very considerable experience in this field. The text is enlivened from time to time with case histories of individual patients whose epilepsy he has managed. A great deal of information and tips of great importance in relation to treatment abound throughout the pages of the volume. I have learned a great deal from reading it and have no doubt that I shall turn to it often in the future for advice relating to the management of individual patients. I am confident that many doctors will find this publication as interesting and useful as I have. It is in my view likely to become an indispensable *vade mecum* for all who treat patients with epilepsy, being full of wise counsel. Doctors and patients alike will in my view find it of inestimable benefit.

SIR JOHN WALTON
Oxford
October 1983

Foreword

The unique approach used in this volume on the diagnosis and treatment of epilepsy is deceiving. At first glance, the work may appear to be little more than a pocketbook of a hundred rules to be followed pedantically. It is much more than that, however. It is a basic source of well-referenced information about epilepsy for an audience ranging from medical students to experienced epileptologists. The former will appreciate its instructive approach and the latter will draw on the principles in formulating treatment plans for patients with epilepsy. These are essentially guidelines, not procedural dicta. Nevertheless, certain basic principles are crucial to the effective medical management of seizures. This volume offers a very personal but well-balanced interpretation of these principles. It also touches upon the no less important psychological concerns of epilepsy and explores the promising research advances that hold hope for improved care of persons with epilepsy.

Both students of epilepsy and clinicians working with epileptic patients have in this monograph a well-refined, practical treatise on the essential elements of the diagnosis and treatment of epilepsy. There is no better qualified author of this subject than Dr. Porter.

J. KIFFIN PENRY
Winston-Salem, N. C.
June 1983

Preface

In the course of evaluating and treating patients with epilepsy, I have often observed that many mistakes could be avoided if certain diagnostic and therapeutic principles were known to the physician. Although a careful review of other books on epilepsy revealed many important principles, I was determined to choose my own and condense them to stress those most important to me. I have assembled 100 principles as a starting point for the medical student and doctor confronted with one of the millions of patients with epilepsy.

The approach is admittedly simplistic, but if the practitioner becomes aware of how epileptologists approach, diagnose, and treat patients, I am confident that better seizure control, fewer adverse side effects of drugs, and improved psychosocial conditions will prevail. Few rules in medicine are immutable, however, and these are no exception. This book represents one neurologist's approach to the management of epilepsy.

The diagnostic sections emphasize adequate seizure classification, especially insofar as it can be derived from the patient's medical history. The terminology is taken from the most recently published classification of epileptic seizures; older terms are also explained. The sections on therapy emphasize nonsedative medications and their proper use. The book is not primarily designed for use in the care of neonates or infants, although many of the principles apply to such patients as well.

Though I am grateful to many for my understanding of neurology and epilepsy, this book is wholly mine; I alone am responsible for both its errors and its possible contribution to the care of people with epilepsy.

Acknowledgments

Of my many mentors, I thank most especially Dr. Robert A. Fishman, who taught me about neurology, and Dr. J. Kiffin Penry, who taught me about epilepsy. I am grateful for the adventuresome spirit and valuable suggestions of Sir John Walton and the guiding hand of Dr. Barend ter Haar of W. B. Saunders Ltd. Drs. William H. Theodore and Philip H. Sheridan made helpful suggestions on the manuscript. The first draft was typed in part by Ms. Pauline Lainas; later drafts were typed on the computer-age invention of Dr. Adam Osborne. Ms. Bettie Jean Hessie has provided editorial assistance to me for more than a decade; I could not have written this book without her extraordinary talent and energy. Finally, I thank my family for their patience, and most especially my wife, Candace, to whom I have dedicated this book.

CHAPTER ONE

Approach to the Patient

1. The brain is just another body organ.

Neurologists, neurosurgeons, and psychiatrists take pride in the domain that makes their specialties unique — the domain that makes man unique: the brain and its connections. Awesome and remarkable though it is, the human brain differs from other animal brains only in the degree of its complexity. Like other body organs, the brain is both vulnerable and resilient; it gets sick and then often recovers. Just as with other body organs, the symptoms of the brain's illness are unique to its function.

It is important for practitioners who deal primarily with the heart, lungs, kidneys, and other body organs to realize that neurologists, neurosurgeons, and psychiatrists do not have a monopoly of understanding the brain. Most primary care physicians (family doctors) should be aware of the fundamentals of diagnosis and therapy in medical neurology. Just as some knowledge of psychiatry is a necessary everyday requisite in the practice of most physicians, a basic understanding of neurology is essential for effective patient care.

Epileptic seizures are but one of the many symptoms of a sick brain. The patient with epilepsy should be viewed as a person with a brain that malfunctions intermittently. The physician should approach the epileptic patient in the same way that he would approach a patient with transient cardiac arrhythmias, that is, with matter-of-fact attention to the diagnostically and therapeutically important details. Although patients with complex problems may require the attention of a specialist, many patients with seizures can be treated by the primary care physician who has a firm grasp of the elementary principles of the diagnosis and management of epilepsy.

2. Assume that every patient with epilepsy wants to get well.

Despite years of frustration , patients with difficult seizure problems are almost always hopeful of discovering something new — a new doctor, a new medication, a new procedure — that will enable them to lead a normal life. Although the physician must carefully temper his optimism about any new therapy, most patients are willing to try a new regimen in the hope of achieving better seizure control. It is, therefore, incumbent on the physician to offer the best possible therapy. Improvements lost while trying a new regimen are

1

usually regained by returning to the former treatment program, if the new regimen is a failure; thus the fear of trying something new should be allayed. Although the practitioner must be especially wary of the possibility of life-threatening generalized tonic-clonic status epilepticus when a new regimen is introduced, such an event is almost always avoidable if therapeutic plasma levels of phenytoin and/or carbamazepine are maintained and if changes are not made too rapidly.

Patients with severe seizures naturally become depressed when neither renewed hope nor new approaches are offered. There are indeed many patients who have uncontrolled seizures, but they deserve thorough evaluation in a referral center before their condition is considered refractory.

3.   Concealing the diagnosis usually causes more harm than it avoids.

In a small and fortunately diminishing number of patients, the family may be advised not to tell the patient, usually a child, the correct diagnosis, that is, seizures or epilepsy. Clearly, patients who have epilepsy must be considered individually, but most affected individuals are much better off if they are given an early explanation of both the nature of the disorder and the potential prejudices that they may encounter in society. If secrecy is attempted, the whole family must 'live a lie,' with constant fear that the truth will suddenly emerge; this fear may shatter the patient psychologically. The resulting pressure on the family can be so severe that the patient suffers greater harm from the secret-keeping process than the truth would ever have caused. Furthermore, the patient's ignorance of the truth can damage the relationship between the patient and his doctor (Riley, 1980).

4.   Attack the problem with vigor.

Armed with the knowledge that many seizure problems are controllable and that most patients are willing to try new approaches, the physician should not hesitate to attack the problem with vigor. Just as with any other disorder, the physician needs to (1) establish the diagnosis, (2) set a therapeutic goal, (3) define the best and safest plan to reach this goal, and (4) proceed with the plan. If the patients are seen frequently and if appropriate changes are made slowly and deliberately, very few are likely to experience more than a slight increase in seizure frequency during medication changes.

5.   Refer patients with refractory epilepsy to a comprehensive epilepsy center.

Every patient with uncontrolled epilepsy should have the satisfaction of knowing that all measures capable of producing improvement have been exhausted. Although most diagnostic and therapeutic possibilities can be adequately evaluated by the primary care physician or neurologist, specialized investigation and management can occasionally lead to revision of the diagnosis of epilepsy, a better pharmacologic regimen, or the use of surgical therapy; a dramatic improvement may be the result.

There are several kinds of comprehensive epilepsy centers. In the United States, for example, the Comprehensive Epilepsy Programs of the National Institutes of Health (NIH) are not only involved in clinical research but also have capabilities for extensive inpatient evaluation. All NIH programs will also offer outpatient opinions. The U.S. Veterans Administration Epilepsy Centers treat veterans; some also treat nonveterans. There are other outstanding clinics and university centers in the United States to which appropriate referrals can be made. The best way to be certain of the expertise available in a particular area of this country is to write to the Epilepsy Foundation of America, 4351 Garden City Drive (Suite 406), Landover, Maryland 20785 U.S.A.

The United States, however, is less advanced in the comprehensive care of epilepsy than many other countries, in which long-term comprehensive care is available in nationally funded centers. Such centers emphasize not only the need for long-term hospitalization for proper evaluation and treatment of epilepsy but also the need for eventual deinstitutionalization to the maximum extent possible. In addition to such centers, there are many outstanding clinics and hospitals throughout the world in which patients with refractory seizures can be definitively evaluated. Information on the location of specialized epilepsy centers and clinics can be obtained from the national or local voluntary or professional epilepsy society. The addresses of the local societies around the world are available from Epilepsy International, Via G. Gozzi 1, 20129 Milan, Italy. The national chapters of the International League Against Epilepsy and the International Bureau for Epilepsy are listed in the Appendix.

CHAPTER TWO

Diagnosis: Causes of Epilepsy

6. There are two levels of diagnosis in every patient with epileptic seizures; both are important.

At a fundamental level, the *etiologic diagnosis* involves identification of the cause of the epileptic seizures. At a more superficial yet therapeutically important level, the *seizure diagnosis* is based on the nature of the seizure type. The search for both diagnoses is necessary for the proper care of the patient with epilepsy. Failure to establish the etiologic diagnosis means that some patients will continue to have seizures because of, for example, undiagnosed tumors. Failure to establish the seizure diagnosis means that some patients will continue to have seizures because, for example, absence attacks have been treated as complex partial seizures. This is not to say that there is no relationship between the etiologic diagnosis, which is often unknown, and the seizure diagnosis, which can almost always be determined. There usually is such a relationship, and knowledge of one may lead to an understanding of the other.

To understand better these two types of diagnoses, one might consider a limited analogy to bacterial pneumonia in a setting of underlying lung cancer. The patient might have pneumococcal or staphylococcal or *Pseudomonas* pneumonia, each requiring a different therapy. Treating the pneumonia in this case is much like treating the different types of seizures with different antiepileptic drugs. The patient's fundamental (etiologic) diagnosis, however, is the cancer; the pneumonia is a complication or symptom of the fundamental etiologic problem.

Clearly, it is just as inappropriate to say simply that a patient has seizures without giving a definitive seizure description as it is to say that a patient has pneumonia without naming the responsible organism. Equally important, of course, is the cause of the seizures, although it unfortunately remains unknown in many patients with epilepsy.

7. Both the etiologic diagnosis and the seizure diagnosis can often be obtained from the patient's medical history.

According to Reiser (1978), the reverence of modern clinical medicine for objective evidence — data sensed and generated by machines and interpreted by technicians and specialists — has led to skepticism about the patient's subjective statements and distrust of subjective clinical judgments.

Although objective information plays an increasing role in diagnosis and therapy, the vast storehouse of data, however flawed, that is available directly from the patient must not be overlooked. The experienced physician need not listen to a rambling, disorganized monologue — quite the contrary. There are certain facts critical to the diagnosis of epilepsy that may only be revealed by interrogation. Although every doctor has his own interviewing technique, some questions are indispensable. First, one must obtain a detailed description of the seizures. Many patients are not prepared for this line of questioning; others will give a terminology-oriented description, using such terms as 'petit mal' or 'temporal lobe.' The doctor must reorient the patient to more fundamental, descriptive terms (Porter, 1983a). The doctor may begin by asking the patient, 'What is the first thing that happens in a typical seizure?' Patients with simple partial seizures (or auras) will be able to describe the entire event by themselves in logical sequence. Patients with complex partial seizures will need assistance, either from persons who have seen the attacks or from a knowledge of what they have been told. The doctor may ask, for example, 'What do other people see when you have a seizure? What do they observe?' Finally, it is important to learn whether the attack ends abruptly or whether it tapers into a postictal state. One good question is 'Do you feel bad or tired after an attack?' A positive response strongly suggests the presence of an abnormal postictal state; such attacks are unlikely to be absence attacks, for example (Porter, 1983a).

It is not usually necessary, except when psychogenic seizures are considered in the differential diagnosis, to obtain a detailed description of generalized tonic-clonic (grand mal) seizures; such seizures are rather stereotyped and accompany a wide variety of more fundamental seizure types. They are often secondary to the fundamental seizure type and are relatively easily controlled in most patients.

This history-taking process should, in most cases, lead to the seizure diagnosis (see Chapter 3). The seizure diagnosis may greatly aid in establishing the etiologic diagnosis; determining the seizure type will even tell whether or not the etiology is likely to be uncovered at all. A 10-year-old girl with 35 attacks per day of sudden unresponsiveness, eyelid blinking, and lip smacking, lasting 10 to 15 sec each, followed by instantaneous return to normal mental function, will almost certainly have absence seizures with clonic motion and automatisms (principles 24 to 26); the etiologic diagnosis may remain unknown. A 40-year-old man with daily paroxysmal attacks of a bad odor followed by lip smacking and fumbling and then several minutes of postictal confusion and lethargy has complex partial seizures with a simple partial onset (see Chapter 4); the etiologic diagnosis is tumor until proved otherwise. The medical history is, therefore, invaluable and must receive special emphasis in the diagnosis of patients with epilepsy.

The medical history is easier to obtain if the patient is adequately prepared before the first visit to the physician and is accompanied on this visit by someone who has seen the attacks. The following letter, or a similar one, should be sent to the patient a few weeks before the first visit to the physician. This sample letter is designed especially for referral centers, where long-term intractable epilepsy is commonly seen; the seizure description portion, however, applies to all patients.

LETTER TO PATIENT

Dear (Patient):
You will be evaluated in the epilepsy outpatient clinic on (date). It will be of great help to the examining physician if you can collect the following information prior to this visit:

1. Make a summary of the history of the seizures. Note when they first began, how frequently they occurred, and what types of seizures occurred.
2. Recall whether the nature of the seizures has changed since they first started. Be prepared to describe each type of seizure in detail. Ask people who have seen a seizure to describe it to you.
3. Try to remember the order in which medications were given, dosages changed, and new medicines started.
4. Recall which medicines affected the frequency of your seizures.
5. Recall the exact number of each type of seizure you have had in the past month.
6. If possible, have someone who has witnessed a seizure accompany you to the clinic.

The more precise the information, the better will be our understanding of your problem.

(Doctor's Signature)

8.   There are many etiologies of the epilepsies.

Epilepsy can be caused by virtually all of the serious diseases or disorders of humans. It can result from congenital malformations, infections, tumors, vascular diseases, degenerative diseases, or injury. In more than three-fourths of patients with epilepsy, the seizures begin before the age of 18 years (Commission, 1978). The reason for this age of onset is not clear, but the vulnerability of the developing nervous system to seizure discharge is known clinically and documented experimentally. Any categorization of the causes of epilepsy should, therefore, attempt to distinguish between the causes in children and the causes in adults. Table 8.1 lists, in descending order of probable incidence, the main causes of seizures in children and adults.

In a substantial proportion of patients, the etiology of the seizures remains undetected. Future scientific advances are likely to identify two principal causes of epilepsy in this population. The first of these is inherited susceptibility. Although there is considerable evidence that absence seizures, for example, are an expression of an autosomal dominant gene (Metrakos and Metrakos, 1961), the role of genetic factors in epilepsy is almost wholly unexplored (Newmark and Porter, 1982). Although it is tempting to hold 'genetic predisposition' responsible when a certain patient has epilepsy after a head injury and another, equally injured patient has no seizures, this implication is almost pure speculation. Head injury as an important cause of epilepsy is discussed in principle 97.

The second probable cause of epilepsy in patients with seizures of

Table 8.1. Important causes of seizures in children and adults in order of probable incidence

Infants and Children	Adults
No definite cause determined	No definite cause determined
Birth and neonatal injuries	Vascular lesions
Vascular insults	Head trauma
(other than above)	Drug or alcohol abuse
Congenital or metabolic disorders	Neoplasia
Head injuries	Infection
Infection	Heredity
Neoplasia	
Heredity	

From Porter (1980b).

unknown origin is chronic or subclinical infection. With the identification of various agents that can cause disease without overt evidence of inflammation, such as Creutzfeldt-Jacob disease, and with the observation that many viruses, such as herpes, are present in latent form in humans, the following speculations are possible: (1) persistent viral infection must be considered in any chronic central nervous system (CNS) disease of unknown etiology; (2) the chronic infection may not have an acute phase or may not be accompanied by the systemic signs generally associated with acute encephalitis, such as malaise, fever, or even changes in the cerebrospinal fluid (CSF); and (3) it is likely that many causative agents of persistent infection have not yet been identified (Porter, 1980b).

Finally, it should be noted that the effort to uncover the cause of epilepsy in a patient contributes directly to the etiologic diagnosis, but only indirectly to the seizure diagnosis. Classifications of the epilepsies, based on etiology, are possible (see Table 13.1), but classifications of seizures based on etiology have thus far been unsuccessful.

9. Ascertaining the etiologic diagnosis requires careful judgment in the use of special procedures.

In the investigation of neurologic disease, a hierarchy of laboratory studies has gradually been established to follow the history-taking process and physical examination of the patient; this hierarchy has recently been modified by computer-assisted tomography (CT), which provides invaluable anatomic information with little risk to the patient. A CT scan, however, is not necessary for every patient with seizures. The following four stages of study generally suffice for the proper evaluation of patients with seizures: (1) medical history, neurologic examination, and electroencephalogram (EEG), (2) CT scan, (3) advanced studies, and (4) positron emission tomography (PET).

Stage 1

No patient with seizures deserves less than a complete stage 1 examination. The medical history has been emphasized in principle 7. The neurologic
examination is one of the most specific and revealing of physical examinations.
Properly conducted and interpreted, it may add considerable additional
information. On the other hand, it often reveals no abnormalities in patients
with seizures, especially generalized seizures. The EEG is useful in establishing both the etiologic diagnosis and the seizure diagnosis, and as a dynamic
physiologic tool, its overall importance in evaluating epilepsy remains
undiminished.

A review of either the neurologic examination or the EEG is beyond the
scope and intent of this book. The fundamentals of the neurologic examination are well described by DeJong (1977); basic electroencephalography is
well defined by Kooi et al. (1978), Kiloh et al. (1981), and Klass and Daly
(1979). It should be noted that the neurologic examination and the EEG
usually confirm information revealed by the medical history. The limited
emphasis in this book on the EEG reflects the view that most diagnostic and
therapeutic decisions are made primarily on the basis of information obtained
in this way. The more complicated the case, the greater the need for
electroencephalographic or other laboratory data. Intensive monitoring is
used almost exclusively to establish the seizure diagnosis (principle 18).

An example of a patient who needs only a stage 1 evaluation is a
9-year-old boy with normal intelligence who has 15 to 20 attacks per day of
staring, blinking of the eyelids, lip smacking, and rapid return of normal
consciousness after 10 to 15 sec without postictal lethargy or other sequelae.
His neurologic examination is normal, and his EEG shows 3-Hz generalized
spike-and-wave discharges superimposed on a normal background. No
localizing features are apparent. He has absence seizures, the etiology of
which may remain unknown.

Stage 2

An example of a patient who needs a Stage 2 investigation is a 26-year-old
woman with normal intelligence who has had a recent onset of two attacks a
week of 60 sec of unresponsiveness associated with staring, lip smacking, and
fumbling with her clothing, followed by gradual return of consciousness over a
2-min interval following the initial unresponsiveness; the patient then has
general malaise and fatigue lasting for 30 min. The neurologic examination is
normal, but the EEG demonstrates right anterior temporal spikes. The
seizure diagnosis is clear, that is, complex partial seizures, but a cerebral CT
scan is warranted to establish the etiologic diagnosis.

Although the CT scan represents a somewhat expensive addition to the
investigative armamentarium, it gives extensive and accurate anatomic
information with minimal patient morbidity. It is indicated in virtually every

patient with partial seizures and in most patients with generalized seizures, such as those with generalized tonic-clonic seizures. It may be indicated in other types of generalized seizures, depending on their severity and the degree of associated neurologic abnormality. Many patients with absence seizures do not need a CT scan; other seizure types in which no anatomic lesion is likely to occur may not require such an investigation either.

The use of contrast enhancement allows the detection of a larger number of cerebral abnormalitites by the CT scan. To conserve time and money when the suspicion of a detectable anatomic lesion is only moderate, the CT scan will generally be done only once; the scan should, therefore, include intravenous contrast if it is not contraindicated because of sensitivity to the dye or for other reasons. If an abnormality does appear with contrast, the lesion can be reexamined one or two days later without contrast to gain additional insight into its nature. Allergic reactions to the contrast material must, of course, be anticipated and adequately treated. Impaired renal function (from diabetes, for example) is apparently one relative contraindication (Theerman, 1979).

Stage 3

Further investigation is indicated when the CT scan reveals a lesion but further information is needed for definitive diagnosis or localization, or when the CT scan shows no abnormalities but other evidence strongly suggests a therapeutically approachable lesion.

The most benign of the more advanced studies is lumbar puncture, which permits evaluation of CSF pressure, cellular components, glucose content, and protein fractions. Lumbar puncture should be performed in all patients in whom the etiologic diagnosis is unclear, except those few whose medical history has remained stable and whose previous CSF findings were normal. The main reason for delaying lumbar puncture is increased intracranial pressure, which increases the possibility of herniation. Overall, examination of the CSF allows evaluation of several diagnostic possibilities, many of which cannot be determined by any other tests. The monograph by Fishman (1980) is recommended for further understanding of the usefulness of lumbar puncture and CSF examination.

If either the CT scan or lumbar puncture reveals abnormalities, the type of additional study or studies then indicated is determined by the kind of information needed. For example, if a tumor is apparent or suspected from the CT scan results, arteriography is usually indicated before surgical intervention. In patients with suspected atrophic lesions, pneumoencephalography only rarely delineates the temporal horns more fully than the newest CT scanners. The isotope brain scan, using a radioactive tracer, adds another test of the permeability of the blood-brain barrier, and may verify or contribute to the diagnosis and localization.

When the CT scan shows no abnormalities but the neurologic examination or the EEG findings suggest a lesion, examination of the CSF may be diagnostic. Arteriography or other relatively high-morbidity studies in the presence of normal CT scan results are not often indicated, but the justification for such studies resides in the abnormalities they sometimes reveal. Surgical intervention specifically for epilepsy is one prominent exception; the CT scan results may be normal, but other studies are needed to provide additional anatomic information for the surgeon (principles 90 and 91). Neuropsychologic data, important for many patients with epilepsy, are especially important in the presurgical evaluation.

The echoencephalogram has limited usefulness in the neurologic evaluation of patients with epilepsy. It can define the diencephalic midline in comatose patients, but has been largely supplanted by the much more informative CT scan.

Stage 4

Positron emission computed tomography appears likely to make considerable changes in the evaluation of epileptic patients. It combines the 'slice technique' of the CT scanner with the physiologic advantages of an injectable radioactive tracer, which can be concentrated in areas of altered metabolism or blood flow. If localized changes in the metabolic rate are found, they may greatly assist in the pre-surgical evaluation, especially in patients with partial seizures. The PET technique is available in very few centers; it remains experimental and expensive. Nuclear magnetic resonance (NMR) scanning probably will prove equally informative but less expensive and more widely available (principle 100).

10. Occasionally reevaluate the etiologic diagnosis in patients with intractable seizures.

One pitfall in evaluating patients who have a long history of uncontrolled seizures is to assume that no new information is discoverable. In fact, pathologic lesions may change with time and many become recognizable years after the first seizure. Furthermore, new and improved techniques such as CT scanning improve the likelihood of establishing an etiologic diagnosis. This is especially true for patients with partial seizures, localized EEG abnormalities, or focal neurologic abnormalities on examination. Such patients deserve a complete neurologic reevaluation at least through stage 2 (principle 9) at a minimum of every 3 to 5 years and more frequently if any of these signs worsen.

Two case reports exemplify the problem. The first case illustrates the potential benefits of such a reevaluation. The second unfortunately confirms that, in some patients, seizure control may not be improved even if the etiologic diagnosis is established.

Patient 1

A 33-year-old man had complex partial seizures for 10 years. He was evaluated at the age of 28 years, at which time a CT scan with contrast enhancement was minimally suggestive of a left temporal lobe lesion. The patient's seizures were poorly controlled on maximally tolerated doses of appropriate antiepileptic drugs. Approximately 1 year later, a repeat CT scan was performed, using a different, much improved scanner. A definitive lesion was identified, and a left temporal lobe vascular malformation was removed. The patient has been seizure free for 4 years. He has returned to college and earned a bachelor's degree and is now seeking employment.

Patient 2

A 35-year-old man had complex partial seizures since the age of 15 years. One year after the seizures began, an angiogram revealed a right frontal avascular lesion, thought to be related to a near-fatal strangulation episode at the age of 5 years. The patient had uncontrolled seizures but was not fully reevaluated until the age of 29 years, when the avascular mass was again disclosed by angiography; a low-grade astrocytoma was partially removed. Two subsequent hospital admissions for seizure control were unsuccessful. At age 31 years, another subtotal right frontal lobectomy was performed with 'resection of tumor in the right frontal region and surrounding epileptogenic tissue.' The patient's seizures resumed shortly after discharge with no long-term improvement to date.

11. Sudden, unexplained death remains a serious problem in patients with severe epilepsy.

'The danger to life in epilepsy is not great. Alarming as is the aspect of a severe epileptic fit — imminent as the danger to life appears when the patient is lying senseless, with livid, swollen and distorted features, and convulsions which almost asphyxiate him, looking "as if strangled by the bow of an invisible executioner," it is extremely rare for a patient to die during a fit. The chief danger of death in an attack is the liability to accidental asphyxia, in consequence of the occurrence of an attack during a meal, when food may get into the air-passages, or of vomiting after an attack with the same result, or in consequence of the patient, in bed, after an attack, turning on the face and being suffocated in the post-epileptic insensibility.' Thus did Gowers, in 1885, observe that epileptic seizures are rarely associated with death but that some patients do in fact die, perhaps from various causes of asphyxiation.

Some studies confirm the overall increased incidence of mortality in patients with epilepsy (Hauser et al., 1980), but since the time of Gowers little new knowledge has emerged about the causes of sudden death in patients with epilepsy. Many reports have focused on asphyxia, perhaps because convulsions inherently cause respiratory embarrassment. A case report exemplifies the problem:

A 17-year-old girl was well until one year previously, when she had the sudden onset of viral encephalitis associated with multiple generalized tonic-clonic seizures, confusion, and lethargy for approximately 2 weeks. She was left with a residuum of memory loss and frequent generalized tonic-clonic seizures. A regimen of phenytoin and carbamazepine was gradually prescribed to maximally tolerated doses, and the patient slowly improved. She had returned to special classes in school, and her seizure frequency had decreased from an average of three seizures a week to one or two a month. She was found dead at home by her parents, her face buried in the pillow. An autopsy was consistent with but not diagnostic of asphyxiation.

Many have blamed pillows for suffocation of patients with nocturnal seizures, but proof is difficult to obtain. Those who speculate about this means of suffocation argue that the usual reflexes are not available to ensure an adequate airway after a generalized tonic-clonic seizure. In the postictal state, should the patient, already acidotic from the seizure, have his head buried in a pillow, the usual corrective tachypnea would be impossible, the acidosis would worsen, and fatal cardiac arrhythmia would result. Neurogenic pulmonary edema also has been implicated as a likely cause of sudden, unexplained death in epilepsy (Terrence et al., 1981). It has also been speculated that increased circulating catecholamines cause fatal cardiac arrhythmias in epileptic patients.

Another, better documented cause of death in epilepsy is drowning. Although patients with epilepsy should be encouraged to enjoy a normal life, swimming must continue to be a regulated activity. Patients with epilepsy, especially those who have alteration of consciousness, should use extreme caution when swimming or boating; poor judgment can result in tragedy. Two simple rules can greatly decrease the likelihood of drowning: (1) Never swim, boat, or play near water without a companion who can swim, and (2) wear a life jacket whenever it is possible and reasonable. The jacket should be designed to keep the head above the water.

12. Neonatal seizures are a separate empirical group.

Volpe (1981) has stressed the need for better definition of the various clinical manifestations of seizures in newborns and has recognized the importance of future clinical research in delineation of the precise relations of seizure type to gestational age, etiology, response to therapy, and outcome. Neonatal epileptic seizures differ greatly from seizures in older children or adults. Convulsions are often encountered during the first few weeks of life and are often the presenting manifestation of serious neurologic dysfunction in the newborn (Rose and Lombroso, 1970). For these reasons, neonatal seizures must be considered as a special diagnostic, therapeutic, and prognostic entity.

Only the most rudimentary aspects of neonatal seizures can be addressed in this volume. The most appealing classification of neonatal seizures is that of Volpe (1981), which divides the attacks into five fundamental subgroups (Table 12.1). Although oversimplified, this classification is highly functional (Fenichel, 1980).

According to Volpe (1981), *subtle seizures* are frequently overlooked; they consist of horizontal eye movements and eyelid blinking, oral automatisms, 'pedaling' and similar stereotyped movements, and apneic episodes. *Tonic seizures* resemble either decorticate or decerebrate posturing,

Table 12.1.   Neonatal seizure types

Order of decreasing frequency
1.   Subtle
2.   Generalized tonic
3.   Multifocal clonic
4.   Focal clonic
5.   Myoclonic

From Volpe (1981).

but are associated with diagnostically definitive eye signs, apnea, or clonic jerks. *Multifocal clonic seizures* are migratory clonic jerks without a 'march,' and are seen especially in full-term infants. *Focal clonic seizures* are unusual, and do not always indicate localized injury. *Myoclonic seizures* are also rare, and are bilateral massive myoclonic jerks; some patients later develop typical infantile spasms.

In the 137 patients studied by Rose and Lombroso (1970), hypocalcemia was the most common etiologic factor in such seizures (20%), followed by intracranial birth injury (15%); lesser, but still important, causes were CNS infection, congenital cerebral malformation, perinatal anoxia, postmaturity, hypoglycemia. Volpe (1981), a decade later, noted that 60% of his cases were caused by perinatal asphyxia and 15% were related to intracranial hemorrhage; these findings probably reflect improvements in neonatal metabolic monitoring and control, although Volpe emphasized the presence of concomitant disorders in patients with hypocalcemia and hypoglycemia.

The approach to the newborn with seizures is urgent if the seizures are continuous. The etiology must be sought and seizure control instituted without delay, as there is increasing evidence that the seizures themselves may damage the child's brain. In most patients, rapid loading with phenytoin or phenobarbital will suffice, although diazepam or paraldehyde may be needed in patients with status epilepticus (Fenichel, 1980). Loading doses of 15 to 20 mg/kg of phenytoin or phenobarbital are needed to achieve therapeutic levels in the newborn; furthermore, orally administered phenytoin is not predictably absorbed (Painter et al., 1981).

The prognosis of neonatal seizures, as with many of the epilepsies, is greatly dependent on the underlying etiology.

CHAPTER THREE

Diagnosis: Seizures and Epilepsy

13. The classification of seizures is different from the classification of the epilepsies.

There is a fundamental difference between seizures and the epilepsies. A seizure is a finite event; it has a beginning and an end. Hughlings Jackson, in 1870, stated that a seizure is a 'symptom…an occasional, an excessive and a disorderly discharge of nerve tissue…' (Taylor, 1931). Epilepsy, on the other hand, is a chronic disorder; it is more a group of syndromes than a disease. The World Health Organization (WHO) has stated that epilepsy is 'a chronic brain disorder of various etiologies characterized by recurrent seizures due to excessive discharge of cerebral neurons…' (Gastaut, 1973). A more appropriate term, 'the epilepsies,' has arisen to emphasize the heterogeneity of these symptom-complexes. The classification of the epilepsies has proved much more difficult to devise and decidedly less useful to the practitioner than the classification of seizures.

The classification of the epilepsies depends on our ability to determine some sort of framework of similarity in patients, seizures, or other factors. The earliest and most persistent subdivision is between epilepsy with a recognizable cause (symptomatic) and epilepsy without a recognizable cause (cryptogenic). The cryptogenic group of patients has been gradually getting smaller as diagnostic techniques improve. The terms 'primary epilepsy' (meaning that the etiology is unknown) and 'secondary epilepsy' (meaning that the etiology is clinically identifiable) have also been recommended. *Secondary epilepsy* is quite different from, and should not be confused with, *secondary generalization of seizures*, a completely different concept (principle 23).

The epilepsies can be classified by many other criteria; some of the possibilities are shown in Table 13.1. Other criteria include anatomy-physiology, precipitants, age at onset, sleep-wake cycle, menstrual cycle, and

14

Table 13.1.   Classification of the epilepsies: Five different methods

---

I. Seizure type and EEG

Commmon generalized epilepsy
  Generalized epilepsy
  Grand mal epilepsy
  Generalized tonic epilepsy
  Tonic epilepsy

Petit mal epilepsy
  Pyknolepsy
  Akinetic epilepsy
  Akinetic petit mal epilepsy
  Atonic epilepsy
  Myoclonic epilepsy
  Myoclonic astatic petit
    mal epilepsy
  Myoclonic akinetic epilepsy
  Propulsive petit mal epilepsy
  Petit mal variant epilepsy

Mixed epilepsy

Myoclonus epilepsy
Nongeneralized epilepsy
One-sided generalized epilepsy

Unilateral epilepsy

Partial epilepsy

Focal epilepsy
  Focal (local) sensory epilepsy
  Somatosensory epilepsy
  Focal (local) motor epilepsy

  Jacksonian epilepsy
  Kojevnikov epilepsy
  Epilepsia partialis continua
  Adversive epilepsy

  Gyratory epilepsy

  Epilepsia cursiva

Psychomotor epilepsy

  Psychic epilepsy
  Affective epilepsy
  Automatic epilepsy
  Gelastic epilepsy
  Autonomic epilepsy
  Thermal epilepsy

II. Etiology

Idiopathic epilepsy
  Primary epilepsy
  Genuine epilepsy
  Essential epilepsy
  Functional epilepsy
  Cryptogenic epilepsy
  Congenital (functional)
    epilepsy of maturation
  Metabolic epilepsy

Genetic epilepsy
  Genetic generalized epilepsy
  Hereditary epilepsy
  Familial epilepsy

Symptomatic epilepsy
  Secondary epilepsy
  Focal symptomatic epilepsy
  Nonfocal symptomatic epilepsy
  Acquired epilepsy
  Organic epilepsy
  Residual epilepsy

Alcohol epilepsy
  Alcoholic epilepsy

Posttraumatic epilepsy
  Traumatic epilepsy

Pseudotraumatic epilepsy

Postsurgical epilepsy

Tumor epilepsy
  Tumoral epilepsy

Atherosclerotic epilepsy

Postencephalitic epilepsy

Penicillin epilepsy

Hypocalcemic epilepsy
Hypoglycemic epilepsy
Renal epilepsy
Allergic epilepsy
Gestation epilepsy

Table 13.1. (cont.)

III. Magnitude of seizure

Major epilepsy	Minor epilepsy
Major motor epilepsy	Minor motor epilepsy

IV. Severity and Chronicity

Benign epilepsy	Intractable epilepsy
Malignant epilepsy	Refractory epilepsy
	Chronic epilepsy

V. Body part

Abdominal epilepsy	Visceral epilepsy
Abdominal vegetative epilepsy	
Enteric epilepsy	Interoceptive epilepsy

From Merlis (1972).

epileptic syndromes. The following preliminary classification of the epilepsies was developed from the combined criteria of seizure type and etiology (Merlis, 1970):

I.   Generalized epilepsies (seizures without localized onset)

   1.   Primary generalized epilepsies
      (etiology unknown)
   2.   Secondary generalized epilepsies
      (etiology known or suspected)

II.   Partial epilepsies (seizures with localized onset)
     (etiology known or suspected)

Although interest in modifying and improving the classification of the epilepsies continues, the emphasis in the last decade has been on the reclassification of epileptic *seizures*. Even though the seizure diagnosis is a highly empirical method of determining therapy, and in spite of the limited theoretical basis for its use, it seems likely that this diagnostic approach will remain valid for a long time to come. The reasons for this are twofold. First, epilepsy apparently has several mechanisms, and each mechanism probably relates to but one or two of the various seizure types presently described. Second, an understanding of the basic mechanisms of the epilepsies seems rather far away, at least in respect of an understanding that would have therapeutic implications. For the foreseeable future, therefore, the seizure type is the best information on which to base a therapeutic decision for the symptomatic treatment of epilepsy.

14. Virtually all seizures can be classified as either partial or generalized.

The first international classification of epileptic seizures (Gastaut, 1970) was the product of many years of effort by a group of experts. It has proved very useful, but extensive use of videotape data has afforded improvements in the classification of seizures (Commission on Classification, 1981).

Seizures are fundamentally divided into two groups — partial and generalized. Partial seizures have clinical or electroencephalographic evidence of a local onset, but the word partial does not imply a highly discrete focus; such a focus often does not exist. The abnormal discharge usually arises in a portion of one hemisphere and may spread to the rest of the brain during a seizure. Generalized seizures, however, have no evidence of localized onset — the clinical manifestations and abnormal electrical discharge give no clue to the locus of onset of the abnormality, if indeed such a locus exists.

Partial seizures are divided into three groups: (1) simple partial seizures, (2) complex partial seizures, and (3) partial seizures secondarily generalized. The distinction between simple partial seizures and complex partial seizures is clarified by the observation that neurologic insults that are confined to one hemisphere, such as a unilateral cerebral stroke, generally spare consciousness, whereas bilateral cerebral (or brain stem) involvement causes alteration of consciousness.

Consciousness in this context is defined as responsiveness. If the patient has some decrement in his ability to respond to exogenous stimuli, then responsiveness, and therefore consciousness, is considered be be altered or lost. Obviously, the degree of difficulty of the task presented will, in part, affect the application of this definition to an individual patient. Exceptional patients with discrete lesions may be unresponsive but aware (e.g., with aphasia); in these patients, whose recall of ictal events is normal, consciousness is considered to be intact. Although responsiveness clearly represents a limited view of consciousness, this definition allows clinical utilization of the classification of epileptic seizures, since the ability to respond during a seizure can usually be tested.

Simple partial seizures (SP) are associated with preservation of consciousness and unilateral hemispheric involvement. Complex partial seizures (CP) are associated with alteration or loss of consciousness and bilateral hemispheric involvement (for exceptions see principles 19 and 20). A partial seizure secondarily generalized is a generalized tonic-clonic (GTC) seizure that proceeds directly from either a simple partial seizure or a complex partial seizure (principle 23).

One of the problems with the original international classification of epileptic seizures (Gastaut, 1970) was its failure to provide for *seizure progression*. With partial seizures, for example, there are six possible progressions:

1. A simple partial seizure may exist alone (with preservation of consciousness).

2. A simple partial seizure may progress to a complex partial seizure (with alteration of consciousness).
3. A complex partial seizure may exist alone (with alteration of consciousness at onset).
4. A simple partial seizure may progress to a generalized tonic-clonic seizure (with alteration of consciousness).
5. A complex partial seizure may progress to a generalized tonic-clonic seizure (with alteration of consciousness at onset).
6. A simple partial seizure may progress to a complex partial seizure, which may then progress to a generalized tonic-clonic seizure (with alteration of consciousness).

These possibilities are summarized in Table 14.1.

In patients with partial seizures, this classification is easily applied clinically to the patient's history. If consciousness is preserved throughout the attack, then the seizure is termed simple partial. If consciousness is lost at the onset, then the attack is a complex partial seizure; if the complex partial seizure was preceded by an aura, then the complex partial seizure had a simple partial onset. Any attack may, on occasion, progress to a generalized tonic-clonic seizure.

If there is no evidence of localized onset, then the attack is a generalized seizure. As heterogeneous as the partial seizures are, the generalized seizures are more so. The generalized seizures include (1) generalized tonic-clonic seizures (grand mal), (2) absence seizures (petit mal), (3) infantile spasms (an epileptic syndrome), (4) myoclonic seizures, (5) atonic seizures, (6) clonic seizures, and (7) tonic seizures. These seizures are listed in descending

Table 14.1. Possible progression of partial seizures

Seizure progression	Seizure name
SP	Simple partial seizures
SP→CP	Complex partial seizures (with SP onset)
CP	Complex partial seizures
SP→GTC	Partial seizures secondarily generalized — generalized tonic-clonic seizures
CP→GTC	Partial seizures secondarily generalized — generalized tonic-clonic seizures
SP→CP→GTC	Partial seizures secondarily generalized — generalized tonic-clonic seizures

frequency of occurrence in the average mixed population of epileptic children and adults. Each of these types will be discussed in Chapter 5.

15. Most patients have a limited variety of seizure types.

It is not true that most patients suffer a wide variety of seizure types. In fact, most patients have relatively stereotyped seizure patterns, and careful history-taking will usually reveal the pattern. The absence seizure pattern, for example, remains relatively constant in an individual patient, even though it is heterogeneous among patients (Penry et al., 1975). In any patient with absence seizures, much of the variability in seizure pattern is clearly related to the patient's environment; these differences in seizure pattern, therefore, are not indicative of some new, fundamental alteration in the pattern of the abnormal electrical discharge.

The recognition of seizure progression is necessary for appropriate grouping of the seizure types. Upon questioning a patient about the nature of his attacks, it is common to discover that what at first appear to be several different types of seizures are in fact fragments (or variants) of a single seizure type. A good medical history will establish the possible progression of one kind of attack to another; a single type of attack may appear to be a variety of attacks to the patient because of its fragmented presentation and because different fragments of the seizure occur at different times.

Although most patients have a basic seizure type, with variations, a few will have a genuinely wide repertory of attacks. For example, the Lennox-Gastaut syndrome (principle 33) is characterized by a variety of seizures in an individual patient. A carefully taken history, however, will usually allow clustering of the seizures into only two or three types.

Another exception to the limited variety in seizure types occurs in the many patients who have generalized tonic-clonic seizures in addition to their fundamental seizure type; these generalized tonic-clonic seizures are often secondary to the fundamental seizure type, but must obviously be classified and treated separately.

16. The postictal state gives many clues to the seizure diagnosis.

The patient with seizures is often momentarily incapacitated by his attack. Some patients are incapacitated further by an abnormal state following the seizure; the occurrence of an abnormal postictal state depends on the seizure type and may be helpful in making the seizure diagnosis. The postictal abnormality may be localized, with minimal disability, or bilateral, with prominent disability. The presence or absence of postictal abnormalities in some of the more common seizure types is shown in Table 16.1.

The implications of the postictal state are especially important in the differential diagnosis of absence seizures and complex partial seizures (principle 26). In a study of 108 videotaped complex partial seizures, distinct

Table 16.1.   Postictal abnormalities in common seizure types

Seizure type	Postictal abnormality
Partial	
Simple partial	Unusual; localized if present
Complex partial	Almost always present, usually as confusion and/or malaise
Secondarily generalized partial seizures	Usually severe, with coma, stupor, confusion, or malaise
Generalized	
Absence	Almost never present
Generalized tonic-clonic	Usually severe, with coma, stupor, confusion, or malaise
Atonic	Varies; may be absent
Clonic	Almost never present

ictal and postictal phases were distinguished in 84%, and the mean postictal duration was 69 sec (range, 3 sec to >7min); only six of the seizures (5.5%) ended abruptly without postictal symptoms (Theodore et al.,1981, 1983a.). Patients with absence attacks, however, have an instantaneous return to normal consciousness following most of their seizures.

17.   Occasionally reevaluate the seizure diagnosis in patients with intractable seizures.

In most patients in whom a thorough medical history has been obtained, the seizure diagnosis will not be in doubt, and therapy can be specifically directed to the seizure type. In some patients, only intensive monitoring will provide the correct seizure diagnosis (principle 18). Patients with intractable seizures must have repeated evaluation of both the etiologic diagnosis and the seizure diagnosis. Clearly, many intractable seizure patients will not respond to any available therapy; this is a challenge for investigators in epilepsy research (Porter, 1983c). On the other hand, long-continued misdiagnosis of the seizure type may also cause therapeutic unresponsiveness and will give a false impression of intractability. The following are two rather diverse examples of misdiagnosis of the seizure type; intensive monitoring aided in the correct diagnosis of each.

Patient 1

The patient was first seen by a referring physician in July 1973, when she was 4 years old. Her spells, in which she previously 'blanked out' for 15 to 20 sec, had changed; she now wandered aimlessly if the seizure began while she was standing. She was seldom confused after the episode. A diagnosis of complex partial seizures was made, and she was given phenobarbital (60 mg/day) and phenytoin (100 mg/day). Her seizures lessened slightly in frequency, but she became drowsy; chloral hydrate was added to the regimen. At age 7 years, she began having temper tantrums, and her mother discontinued all medications. At age 8 years, however, the seizures were so frequent that the child's teacher recommended treatment; phenobarbital, phenytoin, and chloral hydrate were reinstituted. Seizure control was poor, and 6 months later carbamazepine was added; valproate was added 4 months after the carbamazepine.

The patient was seen in a clinic specializing in epilepsy, at which time she was drowsy, inattentive, doing poorly in school, and having 50 seizures a day. It was also evident that she was having absence seizures, not complex partial seizures. A plan of decreasing the phenobarbital and phenytoin, with simultaneous increases in valproate, was undertaken. Within 6 months, she was taking phenytoin, carbamazepine, and valproate, and was having only one or two seizures a week. Within 9 months, she was taking only valproate (1,500 mg/day) and was seizure free.

Patient 2

A 21-year-old woman was well until the age of 13 years, when she began having fainting spells. She was evaluated at a well-known clinic, and although no diagnosis was established, diazepam and phenobarbital were prescribed; the attacks were not disabling. At age 18 years, she began to have attacks, lasting 1 to 2 min, of rigid extension of her body and limbs, with banging of her head backwards, followed by movements of her limbs and postictal confusion; these attacks increased to three a week. She was given phenytoin, mephenytoin, primidone, ethosuximide, and phenobarbital, in various combinations. A pneumoencephalogram, performed at age 19 years, showed no abnormalities. Skull radiographs, brain scan, and EEGs (awake and asleep) gave normal results. Several suicide attempts occurred.

The patient was admitted to an intensive monitoring unit. Psychogenic seizures were diagnosed, and mephenytoin and primidone were cautiously withdrawn. No epileptic attacks occurred. The psychogenic attacks gradually decreased in frequency, and 1 year later they had stopped.

These two case reports emphasize the need to reevaluate the seizure diagnosis in patients in whom a definitive seizure diagnosis is not established, or in those who do not respond satisfactorily to drug therapy. The first patient suffered years of needless epileptic seizures. In the second patient, painful and potentially dangerous studies were performed — studies that intensive monitoring (principle 18) could have obviated if accomplished earlier in her course.

18. Intensive monitoring is sometimes necessary to establish a seizure diagnosis.

When the data on seizure characteristics are inadequate, the seizure diagnosis will be in doubt. If the physician is thereby forced to make a tentative diagnosis, an erroneous decision can result in inappropriate therapy. Even if the seizure diagnosis is correct, multiple medications may be unnecessarily prescribed or plasma drug levels may be inadequate. Intensive monitoring is an extension of the physician's usual skills; it allows more rational diagnostic and therapeutic decisions in the approximately 5% of patients with epilepsy who fail to respond to conventional approaches (Penry and Porter, 1977).

In recent years, there has been an increased interest in all types of monitoring devices. Although monitoring of the vital functions of critically ill patients has been the most dramatic development in this area, advanced techniques of monitoring patients with epilepsy have also emerged. Advances have occurred in EEG monitoring (Porter et al., 1971; Ives et al., 1976; Porter et al., 1976; Porter, 1980a) and in video recording of epileptic and nonepileptic seizures (Penry and Dreifuss, 1969; Penry et al., 1975; Desai et al., 1982). Simultaneous EEG and video recordings have been combined with intensive pharmacologic monitoring in intractable epilepsy (Porter et al., 1977).

Prolonged monitoring of the EEG is not new. Many clinicians and investigators have advocated a departure from the routine 20-min recording, and good laboratories are as flexible with the amount of recording time as they are with modification of montages. Prolongation of a routine EEG recording, however, has the limitations and disadvantages of an artificial environment, confined observation space, prominent artifact if the patient moves about, electrode problems, and excessive accumulation of paper records. In order to collect long-term EEG data for quantification, classification, and localization, two acceptable alternatives have been devised to alleviate these problems. The first is cable telemetry, in which the weak scalp signals are preamplified and then transmitted through a long cable to the EEG machine. The second is radiotelemetry, in which the signal is transmitted by FM radio signal to a receiver and then to the EEG machine. Both systems are effective.

Intensive monitoring with video recording is a more recent advance than EEG monitoring, but it has added an important dimension to our understanding of seizures. There are three basic elements to any video system: cameras, tape recorders, and video monitors. Although integrated systems are available, the best systems are of modular construction, utilizing the best model and manufacturer for each piece of equipment. Adequate technical staff is needed to maintain the equipment in working order. For further discussion of the technical aspects of video recording of seizures, see the various sources cited.

Simultaneous video and EEG recording has been combined with frequent monitoring of antiepileptic drug levels with encouraging results in patients with intractable seizures (Porter et al., 1977). Further, in a study of 69 patients followed for 2 years after intensive monitoring, 58% had improved seizure control, 58% had also maintained a reduction in medication toxicity, and 39% had attained improvement in social adjustment (Porter et al., 1981). In a larger study of 388 intensively monitored patients, severe epilepsy was documented in 267. Improvement in seizure control was effected in 68% of this group; most of the remaining patients had nonepileptic seizures (Mattson, 1980).

Intensive monitoring units have proliferated throughout the world. Although 29 units were estimated to be in place in the United States in August 1980 (Porter et al., 1981), many more have since been built, both in the United States and in other countries.

Long-term ambulatory EEG monitoring without video recording is now possible because of advances in miniaturization of various electronic components (Sato et al., 1976b). The wearable cassette EEG recording device can be used as an aid to diagnosis as well as to quantify electrographic discharges.

CHAPTER FOUR

Diagnosis: Partial Seizures

19. Simple partial seizures are not associated with loss of consciousness.

Simple partial seizures are the most localized of the partial seizures. The discharge is usually confined to a single hemisphere, and the symptoms are specific to the affected brain region. It is the failure of the discharge to spread throughout the brain that explains the sparing of consciousness (see principle 14 for the definition of consciousness).

The new international classification of seizures (Commission on Classification, 1981) lists four main groups of simple partial seizures: (1) simple partial seizures with motor signs, (2) simple partial seizures with sensory symptoms, (3) simple partial seizures with autonomic symptoms or signs, and (4) simple partial seizures with psychic symptoms. The seizures in group 1, focal motor attacks, and group 2, specifically, the sensation of foul odor or taste, are the most commonly observed types.

An aura is nothing more than a simple partial seizure. The word aura (from the Greek, meaning 'breeze') traditionally has been used in epilepsy to refer to the onset of a seizure which the patient is able to describe because he is conscious during the event. The seizure that follows the aura, again from tradition, is usually associated with alteration of consciousness and is usually a complex partial or generalized tonic-clonic seizure. There is nothing fundamentally erroneous about this description, but a broader view is now possible. First, the aura often does not progress further; the aura itself is the seizure. Second, since consciousness is preserved during an aura, and only a small part of the brain is involved, the attack is, by definition, a simple partial seizure. Any partial seizure may progress to another seizure type, and an aura is just one kind of simple partial seizure. A simple partial seizure may precede either a complex partial seizure or a generalized tonic-clonic seizure (see Table 14.1). This progression is apparent to those who treat many patients with partial seizures; treatment often decreases the frequency of the secondary attacks but leaves the patient with the simple partial seizures (auras).

A special type of simple partial seizure with motor signs is that in which spread occurs 'to contiguous cortical areas producing a sequential involvement of body parts in an epileptic march' (Commission on Classification, 1981). Hughlings Jackson contributed to the understanding of such seizures and referred to them as 'cortical epilepsy.' Charcot, however, is credited with popularizing the term 'Jacksonian seizure' for the simple partial motor seizure which 'marches' along the cortex and body parts (Kelly, 1939).

The occurrence of psychic symptoms as the sole manifestation of a simple partial seizure is uncommon but noteworthy. For many years, any seizure characterized by higher cortical dysfunction was described as 'psychomotor' or 'temporal lobe,' independent of the patient's state of consciousness. With video recording, it is clear that some patients can have seizures characterized by paroxysmal symptoms such as *déjà vu,* forced thinking, or overwhelming fear, without alteration of consciousness. These attacks come from localized discharges and deserve to be called simple partial seizures; the new 1981 classification of seizures allows for this rather unusual possibility.

Finally, although the vast majority of simple partial seizures have only unilateral hemispheric involvement, very rarely a simple partial seizure will involve *both* hemispheres simultaneously with sparing of consciousness (Weinberger and Lusins, 1973). These seizures apparently occur because of an abnormal bilateral discharge of limited extent. A recent example recorded on video tape was of a patient who had twitching of the left face and right arm simultaneously, with normal communication during the attack. One might call such an attack a 'bilateral simple partial seizure.'

The prognosis of simple partial seizures is exceedingly variable and is mostly dependent on the etiology. A small cortical venous malformation that causes contralateral focal motor signs may be surgically correctable with minimal deficit. A gustatory or olfactory simple partial seizure is often a premonitory sign of a frontal glioma; the prognosis may be poor. Some patients have continuous simple partial seizures (epilepsia partialis continua), which are often unresponsive to either medical or surgical therapy. One subgroup of simple partial seizures, called variously benign focal epilepsy of childhood, Sylvian seizures (Lombroso, 1967), or Rolandic epilepsy, has a favorable prognosis with or without treatment (Beaussart & Faou, 1978); the seizures usually cease by the early teens. The patients have facial involvement, either somatosensory or clonic jerking, and the seizures usually occur during sleep. The EEG demonstrates central spikes or sharp waves.

The temporary weakness or paralysis (Todd's paralysis) that sometimes follows simple partial seizures is more likely to be caused by active inhibition of neuronal function than by 'neuronal exhaustion'; in this regard one cannot discern ictal from postictal paralysis with any certainty (Efron, 1961).

20. Complex partial seizures are always associated with loss of consciousness.

Complex partial seizures are the most common refractory seizure type in adults. The seizure begins as a localized discharge, but in cases where consciousness is lost at the onset of the attack (i.e., not preceded by a simple partial attack), bilateral hemispheric involvement occurs extremely rapidly. Complex partial seizures are often referred to as temporal lobe seizures or psychomotor seizures. In most patients, the discharges arise in one temporal lobe, but in a few others, they may come from the frontal lobe or other areas, and even though the psyche is always involved, not all such seizures have motor manifestations. Automatisms may occur in complex (but not simple) partial seizures (principle 25). A complex partial seizure may begin with alteration of consciousness or it may be preceded by a simple partial seizure (aura); it may be followed by a secondarily generalized tonic-clonic seizure.

There is some important dissent regarding the thesis that bilateral hemispheric involvement is necessary for alteration of consciousness. Gloor et al.(1980) evaluated 69 complex partial seizures and found 'no evidence for bilateral spread' of the discharge in 19, using depth EEG recordings. They concluded that 'bilateral spread is not a necessary prerequisite for the occurrence of loss of consciousness.' They noted, however, that bilateral spread is the most common feature seen with loss of consciousness and that the mechanism of unilaterally induced loss of consciousness is unknown. This sophisticated study attempted to prove the non-existence of an electrical discharge in part of the brain by inference from depth electrode recordings; the degree of uncertainty attached to such inferences is unknown.

Other characteristics of complex partial seizures have been described by Theodore et al. (1981, 1983a), who found that the duration of the attacks in their patients ranged from 11 sec to almost 8 min (mean, 2 min). Automatisms occurred in 96% of the seizures. Only seven seizures were preceded by auras. Escueta et al. (1977) studied 76 seizures in 14 patients; there were two groups: (1) patients with an initial motionless stare, and (2) patients with automatisms at the onset of the seizure. The latter group may be less responsive to temporal lobectomy, as noted in the further study of 691 complex partial seizures in 79 patients (Delgado-Escueta et al., 1981a).

Differentiation of transient cerebral ischemia from simple partial seizures is usually not difficult; when consciousness is altered during the attack, however, the differential diagnosis between cerebral ischemia and complex partial seizures may not be easy. The former usually occur in older, susceptible persons, and repeated attacks may produce a persistent deficit. Transient ischemia usually lasts longer than most seizures, and the duration of the attack may be the most useful differentiating feature.

The prognosis for seizure control in patients with complex partial seizures is often poor, even in patients whose etiologic diagnosis appears not to be life threatening. Better medical and surgical therapies are greatly needed for this seizure type.

21. By definition, epileptic automatisms can only occur when consciousness is altered.

Automatisms are highly integrated, complex behavioral acts occurring during seizures, of which the patient has no recollection and during which responsiveness is altered (principle 14). Another term for automatisms is automatic behavior. Automatisms include lip smacking, fumbling of the hands, shuffling of the feet, and walking. Any act occurring during an epileptic seizure that requires integration of high-level cortical function may be considered automatic, provided that consciousness is altered.

Automatisms are relatively nonspecific; they occur in both generalized seizures and partial seizures and are apparently determined as much by influences outside the brain as by those within the brain. The nature of the automatism is often determined, therefore, by the patient's environment, either internal or external. A highly detailed classification of automatisms may be found in the work by Penry and Dreifuss (1969); this classification can be simplified into three subgroups:

1. *De novo automatisms from internal stimuli* (including 'release' phenomena), for example, chewing, lip smacking, swallowing, scratching, rubbing, picking, fumbling, running, and disrobing.
2. *De novo automatisms from external stimuli*, for example, responding to pin prick, drinking from a cup, chewing gum placed in the mouth, and pushing in response to restraint.
3. *Perseverative automatisms* (the continuation of any complex act initiated prior to loss of consciousness), for example, chewing food, using fork or spoon, drinking, and walking.

Whether the observed automatisms are ictal or postictal can, in some seizures, be difficult to determine. In absence seizures, all automatisms are ictal because there is no abnormal postictal state. In complex partial seizures, both ictal and postictal automatisms may be observed, but the exact onset of the postictal state itself may be difficult to define. Data are now available on the nature of automatisms in absence seizures (Penry et al., 1975) and complex partial seizures (Escueta et al. 1977; Theodore et al., 1981, 1983a). The data are more complete for absence seizures (principle 25) than for the relatively heterogeneous complex partial seizures (principle 20). The full spectrum of the latter includes such characteristics as formed hallucinations, illusions, affective symptoms, and cognitive symptoms (all during altered consciousness); these have been well reviewed by Daly (1975). The relationship of violent behavior to epilepsy, especially complex partial seizures, is discussed in principle 42.

22. Psychic phenomena may not be helpful in the diagnosis of epilepsy.

Hughlings Jackson (1888) wrote a great deal about alterations of consciousness, especially about partial alterations in epileptic patients who had psychic phenomena during their attacks. He was fully cognizant, however, of the pitfalls of overdiagnosing epilepsy from such data, as he wrote: 'I should never...diagnose epilepsy from the paroxysmal occurrence of 'reminiscence' without other symptoms, although I should suspect epilepsy, if that superpositive mental state began to occur very frequently....' Nevertheless, a tendency remains to consider such phenomena as *déjà vu* as highly suggestive of an epileptic discharge. Harper and Roth (1962) evaluated the frequency of 'temporal lobe' symptomatology in 30 patients with phobic-anxiety (principle 39) and compared the occurrence of these symptoms to that in 30 patients with complex partial seizures. The results are shown in Table 22.1.

Notable is the observation that the symptoms of derealization and 'loss of feeling of familiarity' are actually more common in the phobic-anxiety syndrome than in patients with complex partial seizures (termed 'temporal lobe epilepsy' by the authors, usage consistent with the date of publication). None of the above symptoms, so often thought to be characteristic of complex partial seizures, are more common in patients with epilepsy than in patients with psychiatric problems. The diagnostic value of such phenomena are, therefore, clearly in doubt. If the patient indeed has epilepsy and if consciousness is preserved with such symptomology, the attacks are best classified as simple partial seizures to designate the localized nature of the abnormal discharge (principle 19).

One can apply certain criteria, however, in an attempt to establish which phenomena are most likely to be suggestive of epilepsy. Sensations tend to be more vivid, more stable, and more stereotyped in patients with epilepsy. Although short, paroxysmal symptoms were noted in Harper and Roth's study in both the phobic-anxiety group and the epileptic group, psychic phenomena were usually long lasting in the phobic group but not in the epileptic group; the occurrence of such symptoms for many minutes or even hours suggested that the symptoms were not epileptic in nature. Often, patients with epilepsy had

Table 22.1. 'Temporal lobe' symptomatology in epileptic and nonepileptic patients

	Phobic anxiety syndrome	Complex partial seizures	Statistical difference
Depersonalization	17	11	N.S.
Derealization	11	0	$p<0.01$
Loss of feeling of familiarity (*jamais vu*)	9	1	$p<0.02$
Déjà vu sensation	12	7	N.S.
Formed hallucinations (visual, auditory, olfactory)	11	4	N.S.
Illusions and distortions of perception, including body image changes	12	7	N.S.
Idea of a 'presence'	14	7	N.S.

Modified from Harper and Roth (1962).

psychic symptoms only in association with other epileptic phenomena, such as strange feelings in the stomach (Harper and Roth, 1962).

In summary, the use of psychic symptoms to support the diagnosis of epilepsy is often inappropriate; in virtually all patients other corroborative data are essential to the establishment of the diagnosis.

CHAPTER FIVE

Diagnosis: Generalized Seizures

23. Most generalized tonic-clonic (grand mal) seizures are secondary to another seizure type.

The prevalence of *primary* generalized tonic-clonic seizures has been overemphasized. In point of fact, most generalized tonic-clonic seizures occur secondarily to a less dramatic seizure type. Video recordings of secondary generalized tonic-clonic seizures abound, but recordings of primary generalized tonic-clonic seizures are rare; such primary attacks are probably most common in drug (including alcohol) withdrawal. It is also common to elicit a medical history of the progression of partial seizures to generalized tonic-clonic seizures (principle 14); most, if not all, of the generalized attacks appear to be secondarily induced. Similar observations can be confirmed in generalized seizures. For example, progression of absence seizures to generalized tonic-clonic seizures has been documented clinically and electrographically (Niedermeyer, 1976), and progression of clonic seizures to generalized tonic-clonic seizures has been noted (Porter and Sato, 1982).

Since seizures of both the partial and the generalized categories can progress to generalized tonic-clonic seizures, the latter appear to be a stereotyped expression of maximal involvement of cerebral neurons; this would suggest that the generalized tonic-clonic seizure is the only seizure type worthy of the term 'generalized.' Other seizures in the so-called generalized classification are not truly generalized in the sense of maximal neuronal involvement, but merely have a submaximal bilateral brain involvement. This bilateral involvement, as seen in absence or clonic seizures, for example, may progress to maximal involvement, that is, to secondary generalized tonic-clonic seizures. Unfortunately, such progression is not recognized in the 1981 international classification of seizures; for consistency, this deficiency of the classification will be ignored here. Minor revision of the classification will eventually be necessary to account for this progression.

From the foregoing discussion, it is obviously necessary, in patients with generalized tonic-clonic seizures, to establish the nature of any other seizure type at the time of the initial evaluation, so that appropriate therapy can be instituted for the fundamental seizure type as well as for the tonic-clonic seizures. The stereotyped nature of generalized tonic-clonic seizures as compared with other seizure types makes them relatively easily distinguishable by history. Other seizure types are more subtle and are often more heterogeneous. When taking the medical history, first establish whether or not generalized tonic-clonic seizures are present and are not, for example, psychogenic attacks; then search for a history of other seizure types.

The generalized tonic-clonic seizure is not a random flailing of the body and limbs; it is surprisingly stereotyped, although isolated fragments (principle 15) do occur. The typical attack has been well described by Gastaut and Broughton (1972); tables 23.1 and 23.2 summarize their description.

In addition to the above sequence of events, autonomic changes are prominent. The heart rate and blood pressure may double, and the bladder pressure may increase up to sixfold. Pupillary mydriasis and glandular hypersecretion of the skin and salivary glands occur. Cyanosis of the skin is correlated with the accompanying apnea (Gastaut and Broughton, 1972).

The EEG accompaniments of the generalized tonic-clonic seizure are dramatic but often obscured by muscle artifact. The initial EEG change is usually a desynchronization lasting 1 to 3 sec, followed by 10 sec of 10-Hz spikes; as the clonic phase predominates, the spikes are mixed with slow waves, and finally become a polyspike-and-wave pattern. The EEG is flat, or

Table 23.1. Tonic phase of generalized tonic-clonic seizures

1. Usually lasts from 10 to 20 sec

2. Begins with brief *flexion*:

    (a)   muscles contract

    (b)   the eyelids open; eyes look up

    (c)   the arms are elevated, abducted, and externally rotated; elbows are semiflexed

    (d)   the legs are less involved, but may be flexed

3. *Extension* phase is more prolonged:

    (a)   involves first the back and neck

    (b)   a tonic cry may occur — lasts 2 to 12 seconds

    (c)   the arms extend

    (d)   legs are extended, adducted, and externally rotated

4. The *tremor* begins:

    (a)   the tremor is a repetitive relaxation of the tonic contraction

    (b)   starts at 8/sec, gradually coarsens to 4/sec

    (c)   leads to the clonic phase

From Gastaut and Broughton (1972).

Table 23.2. Clonic phase of generalized tonic-clonic seizures

1. Usually lasts about 30 sec
2. Begins when the muscular relaxations completely interrupt the tonic contraction
3. Brief, violent flexor spasms of the whole body
4. The tongue is often bitten

From Gastaut and Broughton (1972).

nearly flat, after a severe generalized tonic-clonic seizure but gradually recovers to normal rhythms.

The prognosis of generalized tonic-clonic seizures is dependent on all the other factors involved in the patient, especially the etiology of the epilepsy and the other seizure types. In some patients with only idiopathic generalized tonic-clonic seizures, the attacks may prove difficult to control.

24. Absence seizures are well described despite their heterogeneity.

Until the last decade, empirical descriptions of the various seizure types were quite inadequate, and our knowledge of exactly what typifies the various attacks was largely anecdotal. This inadequacy remains for rare seizure types.

The absence (petit mal) seizure was the first to be adequately described. Description was possible because of the high frequency of such attacks in affected children, new techniques of intensive monitoring (principle 18), and an outstanding population of such patients gathered by Dr. F.E. Dreifuss at the University of Virginia. The attacks begin in childhood or early adolescence. Although absence seizures are virtually never reported as beginning after adolescence, certain forms of petit mal status apparently occur in later years as the presenting epileptic symptom (Porter and Penry, 1983).

Prior to the study by Penry and Dreifuss (1969), the absence seizure had been characterized as an attack with a blank stare, motionlessness and unresponsiveness. Although unresponsiveness is the rule, motionlessness occurs in less than 10% of absence attacks; in fact, many other phenomena may accompany such attacks (Penry et al., 1975). Absence seizures are generally brief, usually lasting less than 10 sec and very rarely longer than 45 sec. The attacks are not associated with auras, postictal abnormalities, hallucinations, formed speech, or other symptoms characteristic of partial seizures, generalized tonic-clonic seizures, or infantile spasms. In a video analysis of 374 recorded absence seizures, the attacks were found to be characterized by some combination of the features given in Table 24.1.

There is no difference in the treatment or prognosis of patients with absence seizures who have associated phenomena such as automatisms or clonic motion than in those who do not have such manifestations. Although the likelihood of automatisms in absence attacks increases with the duration of the attack, clonic motion is seen more frequently in the briefer seizures.

Sato et al. (1976a) conducted a follow-up study of 48 patients with

Table 24.1 Features of absence seizures

Feature	Percentage of seizures*
Automatisms	63%
Mild clonic motion (usually eyelids)	46%
Decreased postural tone (usually head nodding)	23%
Increased postural tone (usually arching of the back)	5%
Autonomic phenomena	?

*Many patients had more than one feature.
From Penry et al. (1975).

absence seizures who were initially seen between 1966 and 1968 at the University of Virginia. The follow-up period was 7 years after the initial visit. Multivariate analysis of selected prognostic factors showed that normal or above average intelligence and normal EEG background activity were correlated with improvement. Also prognostically favorable were the absence of concomitant generalized tonic-clonic seizures and a negative family history of seizure disorders. Ninety percent of patients who had all four of these favorable prognostic factors were seizure free at the time of follow-up.

25. Lip smacking does not always mean partial seizures.

Automatisms may occur in generalized seizures as well as in partial seizures. Automatisms are so common in absence seizures, for example, that any seizure longer than 7 sec has more than a 50% chance of having associated automatisms; a seizure longer than 18 sec has a 95% chance of associated automatisms (Fig. 25.1). The commonly occurring automatisms in absence seizures are much the same as in complex partial seizures, although they are apparently somewhat less complicated or prolonged. Lip smacking, chewing, and fumbling of the fingers are commonly observed in absence seizures; less common are swallowing, lip licking, grimacing, yawning, scratching, rubbing, shuffling the legs, walking, and stepping in place. In 374 video-analyzed seizures, automatisms were noted in 236 (63%); almost 90% of patients showed automatisms in at least one attack, but this percentage is conservative, since some patients without evidence of automatisms had only a few attacks recorded (Penry et al., 1975).

26. Mistaking absence seizures for complex partial seizures is the most common diagnostic error leading to inappropriate therapy.

Despite the apparent differences between absence seizures and complex partial seizures, these seizure types are commonly confused. The usual error is to classify an absence seizure as a complex partial seizure, and then to treat the patient with phenytoin and/or phenobarbital, which will control the concomitant generalized tonic-clonic seizures, if present, but will leave the absence seizures uncontrolled. The following example is typical:

> A 24-year-old right-handed man had an 11-year history of uncontrolled attacks characterized by decreased responsiveness lasting less than 10 sec, followed by rapid return to normal consciousness; the attacks occurred many daily. He also had generalized tonic-clonic seizures three or four times a month. He was taking phenytoin (400 mg/day) and primidone (1250 mg/day). The EEG showed bilaterally synchronous 2.5 to 3.5-Hz spike-and-wave discharges on a diffusely slow background. A seizure diagnosis of absence seizures with occasional generalized tonic-clonic attacks was made. The patient was started on valproate, and the primidone was gradually discontinued. His attacks subsided and he has been seizure free for more than 5 years. He is employed and has obtained a driver's license for the first time.

Proper seizure diagnosis is made on the basis of many differential features, but in this patient the most helpful clinical sign was the absence of a postictal abnormality. Confusion, lethargy, or malaise is the rule after most complex partial seizures, but such abnormalities are never present after absence attacks. Occasional complex partial attacks may be followed by instant mental clarity, but the patient will almost always describe other, longer attacks *with* a postictal abnormality; this evidence allows the proper diagnosis. The coexistence of absence seizures and complex partial seizures in the same patient is extremely rare. The therapy and prognosis of these two seizure types is entirely different (principles 20,24,57 and 73).

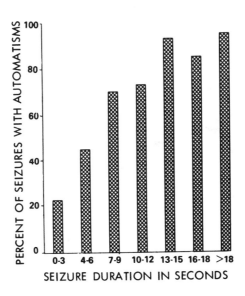

Fig. 25.1. Relation of automatisms to seizure duration in 374 absence seizures. (From Penry et al., 1975.)

27. One-third of all patients with absence seizures also have rarely occurring generalized tonic-clonic seizures.

Sixteen of 48 intensively studied patients with absence seizures also, by history, had generalized tonic-clonic attacks (Penry et al., 1975). It may well be that most of these generalized tonic-clonic seizures were secondary to the absence attacks, but no conclusive supporting data were available (principle 23). The occurrence of generalized tonic-clonic seizures in a patient with absence attacks requires modification of the therapeutic regimen, which is usually different from that of patients who have only absence seizures (principle 79).

28. Not every seizure associated with decreased tone is properly classified as atonic.

Absence seizures are associated, in almost a quarter of the attacks, with some loss of body muscle tone (principle 24). Other seizures, such as simple or complex partial attacks, may also be associated with decreased postural tone. None of these seizures is properly termed atonic. The term 'atonic seizure' is reserved for an especially refractory group of seizures characterized by sudden and precipitous loss of tone. Patients may fall to the floor, often with injury to their head, face, or teeth. During a meal, the patient's head may fall forward into the plate. Helmets, which are a necessity for many of these patients, afford considerable protection, but contribute greatly to the social stigma of epilepsy. Most patients with absence seizures or complex partial seizures do not require helmets because the loss of tone is more gradual — they stumble and stagger but do not fall suddenly; in these attacks the seizure rarely begins with loss of tone. An atonic attack may or may not be followed by a postictal abnormality. Other seizure types are common in patients with atonic seizures.

In early publications on epilepsy, especially of a decade or more ago, a curious use of the term 'akinetic' (without motion) occurred; it came to be synonymous with 'atonic' (without tone). This terminology is especially prevalent in discussions of the Lennox-Gastaut syndrome (principle 33). In the new international classification of epileptic seizures (Commission on Classification, 1981), reference to akinetic seizures has been deleted. There is no evidence for the existence of a separate seizure type characterized only by motionlessness. In fact, many seizure types are characterized by motionlessness, and akinesis is not unique to any group. The preferred term for prominent, sudden loss of tone is atonic. The term 'astatic' (with motion) is also no longer recommended.

29. Myoclonus is a heterogeneous sign and is often a component of a seizure rather than a seizure type.

The terms myoclonus, myoclonic, clonus, and clonic are exceedingly confusing and are used in different ways by virtually all authors. If one assumes that 'clonus' is a 'quick movement,' and that 'myoclonus' is a 'quick movement of muscle,' then the definition of myoclonus given by Marsden et al. (1982) is the simplest and most useful: myoclonus is 'muscle jerking, irregular or rhythmic, arising in the central nervous system.' Logically then, 'clonic' and 'myoclonic' are adjectives derived from the above terms. Unfortunately, common usage often differs from this simple approach.

'Clonus' is most often used to describe the repeated contractions and relaxations, physiologic or pathophysiologic, of the muscle-stretch reflex (e.g., 'sustained clonus at the ankle').

'Clonic' seizures, as defined in the 1981 classification of seizures, are generalized convulsive seizures that are similar to generalized tonic-clonic seizures but lack a tonic phase. Other clonic seizures may be brief generalized attacks that may progress within a few seconds to a generalized tonic-clonic seizure, as may any other epileptic seizure (principles 23 and 34).

'Myoclonic' is often used interchangeably with 'clonic,' especially when used to describe fragments or 'myoclonic components' of a seizure. Myoclonic or clonic components are common in absence seizures, and occasionally even in complex partial seizures. Marsden et al. (1982) have constructed a diagram (Fig. 29.1) in which progressively more severe forms of stimulus-evoked cortical myoclonus are clarified. Not all jerking in response to stimuli is epileptic in origin. Patients with essential startle disease ('hyperekplexia') may simply have an exaggeration of the physiologic reaction of surprise (Gastaut and Villeneuve, 1967).

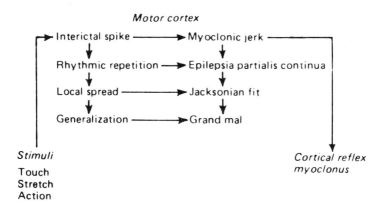

Fig 29.1. Relation of myoclonus to epilepsy. This diagram, which applies to stimulus-induced myoclonus, is useful as a hypothetical model for organizing clinical entities. The diagram is not without its limitations. Most interictal spikes, for example, have no correlation with a myoclonic jerk, and the progression of epilepsia partialis continua is much more often to complete generalization ('grand mal') than to a 'Jacksonian fit.' Nevertheless, the emphasis on the gradual progression from localized and less severe electrographic and clinical entities to more widespread and dramatic events is conceptually correct. (From Marsden et al., 1982)

Many authors refer to 'myoclonus epilepsy' as a specific, progressive syndrome — Unverricht-Lundborg syndrome — which did not, initially, include progressive dementia. Lafora later described a much more malignant form of myoclonus epilepsy with progressive dementia, and, as Marsden et al. (1982) noted, the two disorders became confused. It is common today to divide these genetic syndromes into two groups based on the presence or absence of Lafora bodies in the brain. It is notable that the diagnosis can sometimes be made by liver biopsy (Nishimura et al., 1979) or from other tissues such as skin or muscle.

In contrast to the use of 'myoclonus epilepsy' to describe a severe form of epilepsy, 'myoclonic epilepsy' is often used to describe a benign form of epilepsy (principle 30).

Another well-recognized form of myoclonus is post-anoxic myoclonus, in which lapses of postural control may be as important as the jerking itself (Lance and Adams, 1963). The jerks are brief and occur only with active muscular motion initiated by the patient. This myoclonus may be responsive to specific therapy (principle 82).

Classifications of myoclonus have included anatomic location and etiology (Swanson et al., 1962) and etiology alone (Marsden et al., 1982). In the latter, epileptic myoclonus (Fig. 29.1) is appropriately divided into the fragments of epileptic seizures (e.g., clonic components), and the epilepsies (syndromes with myoclonic seizures as a manifestation). An in-depth discussion of myoclonus is beyond the scope of this book; see the sources cited, the classification of Gastaut (1968), and the monograph by Charleton (1975) for further reading on the subject.

30. Among the clonic (myoclonic) seizure types, there is a benign myoclonic syndrome.

The syndrome of benign adolescent myoclonus is worthy of special note because of the initial fear that the patient may have a fatal disease. In contrast to Unverricht-Lundborg syndrome, it is a rewarding disorder to recognize and treat. It was well described by Boshes & Gibbs (1972). Typically, a teenager or preadolescent child will have the onset of explosive, uncontrollable movements. The jerks will be embarrassing, more frequent in the morning or on arising from sleep, and bothersome at the table when eating. The attacks occasionally progress to generalized tonic-clonic seizures, which may follow directly from an especially severe series of clonic seizures; the tonic-clonic seizures are secondary to the clonic attacks. Valproate is generally considered to be the therapy of choice. Mental retardation does not occur, and the EEG often shows no abnormalities. Attacks worsen with anxiety, sudden stimuli, or sleeplessness. The course is usually one of a few months of worsening, followed by gradual spontaneous improvement. The following is a typical case:

A 15-year-old boy was well except for asthma, when he noticed that he would occasionally drop his spoon or his brush and that his legs would jerk in the morning after awakening. Within a month, his mother noted an outward motion of his arm which knocked a cup across the breakfast table. The jerking became more prominent, with several jerks often occurring in a series; they always occurred, however, within the first 60 to 90 min after arising. A neurologist evaluated the patient but did not prescribe medication. Six months after the onset of the myoclonic jerks, the patient had a generalized tonic-clonic seizure; this attack followed a series of myoclonic jerks and was precipitated by going to bed very late and arising early. The patient was given phenytoin (300 mg/day); valproate was not yet available. The phenytoin dose was later increased to 400 mg/day because of low plasma phenytoin levels. The myoclonic jerks gradually subsided over the following few months and were severe only when the patient was stressed or had inadequate sleep. One year later, he reported having only about two to three jerks a month, and 4 years later he reported having only one or two jerks a year. He has not had another generalized tonic-clonic attack. He graduated from school with his class and at no time showed any signs or symptoms of neurologic disease other than the described seizures.

The largest study of patients with this disorder is by Janz (1957), who described 47 patients. These patients were estimated to represent 3% to 4% of all patients with epilepsy. The usual age at onset of the disorder was between 10 and 23 years, and all but two patients had occasional generalized tonic-clonic seizures in addition to the myoclonic attacks. Janz called the entity 'impulsive petit mal,' in part because of the multispike-wave complex that was found in the EEGs of these patients and that accompanied their attacks.

Halliday (1967) described patients with benign myoclonus who had no other symptoms suggestive of epilepsy and termed the disorder 'familial essential myoclonus.' An autosomal dominant gene is thought to be the mode of inheritance.

31. Onset of spasms before 1 year of age is the rule in 90% of patients with infantile spasms.

Infantile spasms is not a seizure type. It is a syndrome (an epilepsy) encompassing a group of attacks with remarkably diverse etiologies. The recurring attacks, which are brief contractions of the neck, trunk, and extremities, are usually associated with mental retardation and hypsarrhythmia in the EEG. The seizures are usually divided into three different clinical types, although heterogeneity is extraordinary. The following description of each type is taken from the 5,042 recorded seizures reported by Kellaway et al. (1979):

1. *Flexor spasms* are characterized by 'flexion of the neck, arms, and legs' with prominent contraction of the abdominal muscles to 'cause the torso to jack-knife at the waist.' The arms are either abducted or adducted.
2. *Extensor spasms* are characterized by 'extension of the neck and trunk with extensor abduction or adduction of the arms, legs, or both.'
3. *Mixed flexor-extensor spasms* were the most common type, usually with flexion of the body and arms and extension of the legs.

The nature of the attacks has resulted in numerous synonyms for the disorder. According to Lacy and Penry, 1976, some of the synonyms are (1) massive myoclonic jerks, (2) lightning major spasms, (3) flexion spasms, (4) greeting spasms, (5) salaam spasms, (6) jackknife convulsions, (7) infantile myoclonic epilepsy, and (8) Blitz-Nick-Krampfe.

As with many other epileptic syndromes, infantile spasms result from many diverse etiological processes. Lacy and Penry (1976) have identified the most common as (1) idiopathic (approximately 40% of the cases), (2) maternal uterine hemorrhage, (3) maternal toxemia, (4) hydrocephalus, (5) congenital CNS infections (e.g., toxoplasmosis, cytomegalovirus), (6) prematurity (?), (7) low birth weight (?), (8) Aicardi syndrome, (9) perinatal delivery difficulties, (10) kernicterus, (11) trauma, (12) meningitis or encephalitis, (13) immunizations (especially pertussis?), (14) tuberous sclerosis, (15) phenylketonuria and other amino acid abnormalities, (16) neonatal hypo-glycemia, and (17) pyridoxine deficiency (?).

The onset is usually within the first 6 months of life. In the series reported by Charleton (1975), 96% occurred within the first year. The attacks themselves often cluster; the child may have a series of many seizures followed by relative quiescence.

The classic EEG finding, hypsarrhythmia (from the Greek, meaning 'high rhythm'), is seen in most patients, although it is most typical only in the early stages of the disorder (Hrachovy, 1982). When the EEG becomes more organized, as it apparently does with the passage of time, it has been called 'modified hypsarrhythmia.' At least three subgroups of the EEG abnormality have recently been described (Hrachovy,1982), but there is little evidence that such differentiation is useful in predicting the prognosis of the seizures or the associated mental subnormality (Charleton,1975).

The underlying reason for the form of these seizures is unknown. It is intriguing to speculate that the central nervous system has, in its early developmental years, only a limited repertoire of clinical signs and symptoms, and that seizures occuring at this time are more limited in their variability of expression than is the case in adults. Such speculation helps to explain the diverse causes of the syndrome, although it sheds little light on the basic mechanisms of the disorder.

The prognosis of patients with infantile spasms is poor. Of the 214 patients followed at least 3 years by Riikonen (1982), 19.6% had died and only 12% had developed normally. Following cessation of the infantile spasms, more than half the survivors had seizures of a different type, usually partial seizures. Many patients progress to Lennox-Gastaut syndrome (principle 33).

32. Patients with 'mixed seizures' have more than one seizure type.

The term 'mixed seizures' properly refers to a patient with two or more types of classifiable epileptic seizures, such as a combination of generalized tonic-clonic seizures and absence seizures. The term is most often applied to children with Lennox-Gastaut syndrome; these children may indeed have several seizure types, including generalized tonic-clonic seizures, absence seizures, and atonic seizures. From the viewpoints of seizure classification and prognosis, it is important to obtain historical information on the various seizure types individually; only infrequently can this information not be obtained in the course of taking a detailed medical history. In Lennox-Gastaut syndrome, the atonic spells may be much more resistant to therapy and restricting to the patient than the more severe, but more easily controlled generalized tonic-clonic attacks.

Unfortunately, the diagnosis 'mixed seizure disorder' usually implies a paucity of information about the kinds of attacks the patient is having and reflects an inadequate medical history or inability to classify seizures, or both. The same is true for 'minor motor seizure,' which is usually a euphemism for 'small seizure of unknown type, associated with movement.' The latter may refer, for example, to infantile spasms, atonic attacks, absence seizures with mild clonic components, or even simple partial seizures with clonic jerking. The diagnosis of minor motor seizures should be discarded in favor of the proper description of the seizure type.

33. Lennox-Gastaut syndrome is not a seizure type.

'A stare, a jerk, a fall — these represent three seizure phenomena which differ widely in appearance....' Thus did Lennox (1960) set forth his 'petit mal triad,' in which he distinguished three different groups correlated with three different seizure types. The first group is 'pure petit mal' (a stare), which comprises 79% of the triad in Lennox's series, and correlates rather well with what we now call absence seizures (principle 24). Lennox even observed the coexistence of mild clonic motion and automatic behavior with the stare in this seizure type. The second group, 'myoclonia' (a jerk), is admittedly heterogeneous. Lennox divided myoclonias into several subgroups: (1) myoclonic epilepsy, which very roughly correlates to the 'impulsive petit mal' of Janz (principle 30); (2) massive myoclonic jerks, which correlate fairly well with what we now know as infantile spasms (principle 31); (3) myoclonus epilepsy, the progressive syndromes of genetic etiology (principle 29), (4) epilepsia partialis continua, now considered to be a form of continuous simple partial seizures; and (5) palatal myoclonus, a specific myoclonic disorder. Finally, the third group, 'astatic epilepsy' (a fall), correlates best with atonic seizures (principle 28).

Lennox coincidentally made three generalizations about the triad as a whole: (1) the phenomena frequently coexist in individual patients, (2) spike-and-wave abnormalities accompany the attacks, and (3) affected patients have a different response to drugs than do patients with 'convulsions.'

The chief difficulty in accepting the triad was the effort made by Lennox to equate seizure types with epileptic syndromes. Failure to separate the two resulted in confusion for both investigators and practicing physicians. Ironically, Lennox-Gastaut syndrome represents a synthesis of his first unifying observation, that is, that the stare, jerk, and fall frequently coexist in the same patient. This epileptic syndrome was well defined by Gastaut et al. (1966), who described a heterogeneous population of patients with absence, clonic, and atonic seizures. Synonyms of the epileptic syndrome include Lennox syndrome, akinetic petit mal, myoclonic-astatic petit mal, and petit mal variant epilepsy; occasionally the term 'minor motor seizures' is also used to describe the attacks in these patients (principle 32).

Lennox-Gastaut syndrome usually begins between the ages of 1 and 6 years, though rarely it may occur as late as 10 years of age or older. It may develop in patients who have had infantile spasms, but more often occurs spontaneously. The etiologies are diverse. Most patients are mentally retarded. The most devastating seizures are atonic; the head may drop suddenly onto the breakfast table, or the patient may fall precipitously to the floor. Injuries to the face and teeth are common, and helmets are necessary to protect the head. The absence seizures are usually brief, lasting less than 5 sec, and more pronounced tone changes are common. These atypical absence attacks may also have an onset and/or cessation which is not abrupt (Commission on Classification, 1981). Either the atonic or absence attacks may be accompanied by myoclonic jerks. In some cases, the patient appears to be thrown to the floor by the violence of the clonic jerks. The seizures are often severe and intractable. The EEG typically demonstrates 2-Hz spike-and-wave abnormalities, a slower frequency than in typical absence seizures, and the complexes are often irregular and asymmetrical. As the patient gets older, complex partial and generalized tonic-clonic seizures may become predominant.

Some patients appear to have continuous seizures, without remission. One may speculate in these cases that the level of mental function may be due to inadequate numbers of normal neurons, or alternatively, that the available neurons are functioning poorly because of the continuous nature of the widespread discharge. Both factors are likely to be present in most of these patients.

34. Clonic seizures, tonic seizures, or bilateral massive epileptic myoclonus are rare.

Clonic seizures, tonic seizures, and bilateral massive epileptic myoclonus are infrequently seen and will be described only briefly.

Clonic Seizures

Myoclonus is described in detail in principle 29. Noteworthy is a specific type of clonic seizure in which the patient has sudden jerking movements, singly or multiply. The brief attacks may sometimes progress to generalized tonic-clonic seizures. Although some investigators have called such secondary generalization of clonic seizures 'clonic-tonic-clonic seizures,' this is in fact an example of a fundamental seizure type progressing to generalized tonic-clonic seizures (principle 23). The following case exemplifies this seizure type:

> A 30-year-old right-handed man was well until the age of 17 years, when he developed attacks which he characterized as 'shocks,' in which he would suddenly jerk for 1 or 2 sec, with brief alteration of consciousness. He continued to have one to six attacks daily, despite antiepileptic drug therapy. Secondary generalization of the clonic seizures occurred approximately twice a week. Intensive monitoring revealed brief bilateral clonic attacks, especially affecting the arms, with dropping of utensils or cigarettes when an attack occurred. In several attacks, progression to generalized tonic-clonic seizures was recorded. The EEG demonstrated bilateral synchronous spikes and waves. The addition of methsuximide (900 mg/day) caused virtual cessation of seizures, and the patient was discharged on a regimen including this medication.

Tonic Seizures

Not known with certainty is whether the tonic seizure is merely the isolated manifestation of the initial portion of the generalized tonic-clonic attack or whether it is a distinct seizure type. Tonic seizures are common in some patients, but their overall incidence is low. The attack is often severe and is a 'violent, strained distortion of the head, face, and limbs' (Gowers, 1885). The head and eyes deviate, the facial muscles contract, and posturing of the limbs is prominent; the actual posture is variable but most often resembles the posture in the first portion of a generalized tonic-clonic seizure.

Tonic seizures are noteworthy in two syndromes — Lennox-Gastaut syndrome and multiple sclerosis. In the former, Gastaut et al. (1966) noted a 70% incidence of tonic seizures in affected patients. The attacks were occasionally unilateral and sometimes *ended in clonic jerks*. In multiple sclerosis, Matthews (1976) described brief (usually 30 to 90 sec), unilateral attacks of tetanic posture, often sparing the lower extremity; they were frequently painful and often remitted spontaneously. Although an association with epilepsy was noted in only one patient, the tonic attacks appeared to respond favorably to carbamazepine.

Tonic seizures must be carefully distinguished from decorticate or decerebrate posturing. In some patients, especially in infants, this distinction may be difficult (Volpe, 1981). Signs useful in the differentiation include the examination of eye movements, the presence of clonic jerking at the end of some epileptic attacks, and the variable response to antiepileptic drugs.

Bilateral Massive Epileptic Myoclonus

Bilateral massive epileptic myoclonus is an epileptic syndrome and has been deleted from the 1981 classification of epileptic seizures. It will eventually be incorporated into a classification of the epilepsies (principle 13). When described as a seizure type, it is now classified under myoclonic seizures.

The seizures are myoclonic, bilateral, and usually involve all extremities. The attacks vary in importance from the physiologic massive jerk that many experience on falling asleep (not considered epileptic) to the periodic jerking seen in patients with subacute sclerosing panencephalitis. The following case is exemplary:

A 17-year-old boy first became ill in August 1976, with a change in personality. Within 2 months, he noted the onset of occasional jerking in his arms and legs. His schoolwork deteriorated. By November 1976 he was mute and understood only the most rudimentary of commands. The diagnosis of subacute sclerosing panencephalitis was established by measuring high rubeola titers (complement fixation) in both serum and CSF. For several weeks he had, while awake, periodic massive myoclonic jerks occurring every 4 to 8 sec. His condition deteriorated, and he died in late December 1976.

CHAPTER SIX

Diagnosis: Status Epilepticus

35. Convulsive status epilepticus is a medical emergency.

Convulsive (tonic-clonic) status epilepticus is a condition in which the patient has generalized tonic-clonic seizures so frequently that another seizure occurs before the patient returns to normal consciousness from the postictal state; it is a medical emergency with a mortality rate of approximately 10%. It is essential that 'convulsive status [is] stopped as soon as possible...because the molecular events that lead to selective cell death are already operational during the first two to three convulsions' (Delgado-Escueta et al., 1982). Tonic-clonic status is, according to Gastaut (1983), characterized by two types of seizures: primary generalized tonic-clonic attacks or, more frequently, secondarily generalized tonic-clonic seizures following a partial onset. The seizures themselves are typical generalized tonic-clonic seizures (principle 23).

Status epilepticus is usually caused by failure of epileptic patients to take their antiepileptic drugs. Gumnit and Sell (1981) have described the most common causes of noncompliance leading to status epilepticus: (1) The patient may run out of medication and fail to renew the prescription, (2) the patient may take medication only sporadically, (3) the patient may lose the medication and not obtain another supply, (4) the patient, or the physician, may erroneously decide that antiepileptic drugs are no longer needed, or (5) the patient may misunderstand the physician's instructions.

Tonic-clonic status is also more common in patients with known etiologies for their epilepsy (Janz, 1983). The search for the cause of the status epilepticus should therefore be vigorous, especially in older patients. Epileptic patients should also be reevaluated if there is any doubt about the fundamental cause of the status epilepticus. In a series of 2,588 patients with epilepsy, Janz (1983) noted that only 1.6% of 1,885 patients with epilepsy of unknown cause had had a bout of status epilepticus, whereas 9% of patients with epilepsy of known cause had had tonic-clonic status; the most frequent causes of the epilepsy in the latter group were tumor or trauma.

In a study of 98 patients with generalized tonic-clonic status, Aminoff and Simon (1980) noted that, in their urban population, alcohol withdrawal was a major factor in 15 patients; a similar number had cerebrovascular disease as the cause of their status epilepticus. Other causes included intracranial infection, metabolic disorders, drug overdose, and cardiac arrest. In 15% of the patients, no specific cause could be found. Poor outcome correlated primarily with long-lasting status epilepticus. These investigators also noted that the status epilepticus was usually accompanied by hyperthermia and that the leukocyte count increased not only in the peripheral circulation but also in the CSF in 18% of the patients. The special consequences of status epilepticus in infants and children have been reviewed by Aicardi and Chevrie (1983).

Finally, it is important to note that status epilepticus with localizing features suggestive of partial seizures does not always indicate localized pathologic lesions. The phenomenon of partial or lateralized attacks has been asociated in some patients with such diffuse cerebral insults as drug overdose or metabolic disturbance (Aminoff and Simon, 1980). Similar observations have been made in patients with hepatic encephalopathy; localized epileptic seizures do not necessarily mean localized pathologic change (Adams and Foley, 1953).

The therapy of generalized tonic-clonic status is discussed in principle 84.

36. Nonconvulsive status epilepticus is a diagnostic problem.

Although only convulsive (generalized tonic-clonic) status epilepticus is immediately life threatening, the various types of nonconvulsive status epilepticus, such as simple partial status (epilepsia partialis continua), complex partial status (psychomotor status) and petit mal status (spike-wave stupor), are often difficult diagnostic problems. Of the latter groups, petit mal status is the most varied in its nature and form (Porter and Penry, 1983).

Epilepsia partialis continua refers to persistent simple partial seizures, usually with motor manifestations but without a march, and usually remaining confined to the part of the body in which they originated. They may last for hours or days, and although consciousness is preserved, postictal weakness is commonly observed (Commission on Classification, 1981).

Complex partial status is, unlike petit mal status, a *series* of complex partial seizures without intervening return to full responsiveness (Fig. 36.1). The patient's condition cycles back and forth from a deep unresponsiveness during the actual partial seizures to mild-to-moderate alteration between attacks (Porter and Penry, 1983; Treiman and Delgado-Escueta, 1983). Complex partial status is rare, but occurs especially in patients who have severe, intractable complex partial seizures and who have, for some reason, discontinued their antiepileptic medication.

The importance of recognizing and treating complex partial status has been emphasized by Engel et al. (1978) who noted prolonged memory impairment in an 18-year-old girl with four episodes of complex partial status. Treiman and Escueta (1983) also reported persistent short-term memory deficits in two patients with complex partial status. This entity is clearly not benign and requires immediate therapy.

Petit mal status is known by a variety of names. The disorder is exceedingly heterogeneous, and the terminology has been reviewed (Porter

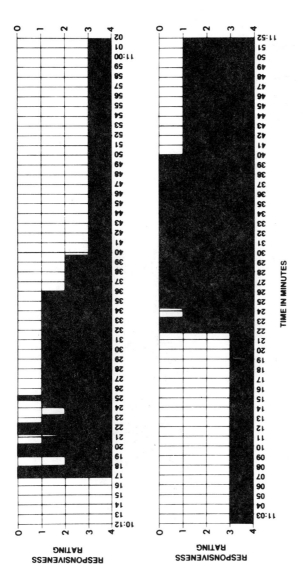

Fig. 36.1. Responsiveness during complex partial status. The patient had a complex partial seizure at 10:17 a.m. and did not recover normal consciousness until several hours later. He had several attacks at the onset of status (10:17 a.m. to 10:25 a.m.), then appeared to be gradually recovering, but had another series of attacks beginning at 11:22 a.m. Recovery occurred gradually. The verbal responsiveness rating is as follows: O = no response; 1 = minimal response; 2 = comprehends, follows simple directions, identifies receptively, cannot answer verbally, anomia may be present; 3 = partial responsiveness, responds appropriately with one or two words and rote phrases, abnormal affect, some anomia; 4 = accurate and immediate response, normal affect, responds to others' comments, and initiates conversation, responds to more than one or two words (From Porter and Penry, 1983.)

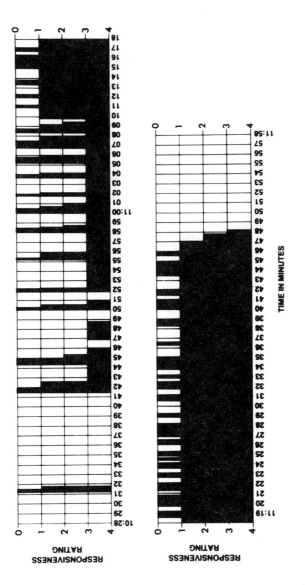

Fig. 36.2. Responsiveness during petit mal status. The patient had a brief absence attack at 10:31 a.m., then a series of attacks beginning at 10:41 a.m., with intervening periods of normal responsiveness. She had severe impairment of responsiveness from 11:10 a.m. to 11:48 a.m., and then made a sudden recovery without postictal abnormality or complaint. The responsiveness rating is the same as in Fig. 36.1 (From Porter and Penry, 1983.)

and Penry, 1983). Only three criteria are applicable to this group of patients, but these are not diagnostic: (1) Continuous (or nearly continuous) epileptiform EEG activity, usually generalized, is found; rarely, only generalized slowing will be noted, (2) behavioral change, usually associated with lethargy and decreased mental function, is present, and (3) there is absence of gross tonic-clonic activity.

The heterogeneity of patients with petit mal status is reflected in the wide variations in ictal EEGs. The classic, more or less continuous, 3-Hz spike-and-wave discharge has been described by many observers, and it probably correlates best with the typical absence seizure — such findings may form a subset of petit mal status and is termed 'absence status.' Other EEG findings include many other spike-and-wave abnormalities, as well as continuous spikes or sharp waves. According to Porter and Penry (1983), 'it is safe to conclude from these data that virtually any generalized, continuous or nearly continuous abnormality could be a substrate for this syndrome.'

The state of altered consciousness may be extremely variable, both inter- and intra-individually (Fig. 36.2). Some patients may be nearly normal, and, according to Andermann & Robb (1972), are 'only aware of a lack of efficiency,' whereas others are barely responsive. Most patients are dull,

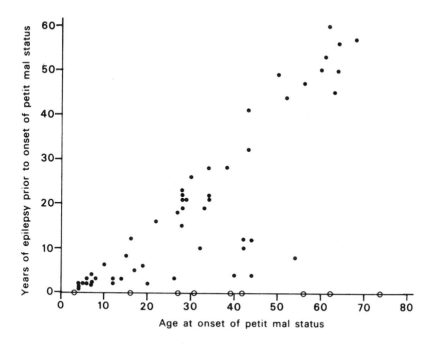

Fig. 36.3. Age at onset of petit mal status in relation to years of preexisting epilepsy. Onset of petit mal status varied from 3 to 74 years of age in 53 patients with epilepsy for <1 to 63 years (*filled circles*). The first bout of petit mal status occurred at ages 3 to 73 in nine patients without a history of epilepsy (*open circles*) (From Porter and Penry, 1983.)

confused, and lethargic; spontaneous activity is decreased. Often, such patients will demonstrate automatic behavior, and may even be able to eat, walk about, or follow simple commands (Porter and Penry, 1983). Mild myoclonia, especially of the eyelids, is also common.

The first attack of petit mal status may come at any age. In some patients, the first attack is the first manifestation of epilepsy. (Fig. 36.3).

Differentiation of petit mal status from complex partial status is important therapeutically, because antiepileptic drug therapy is different for each disorder. The most useful criterion is the medical history, which usually uncovers the underlying seizure type. Another useful criterion is the manner in which the attacks end. Petit mal status usually ends abruptly, without postictal abnormality, even after a prolonged episode, whereas complex partial status is associated with postictal depression, confusion, or malaise. Electroencephalographic data may be decisive in some patients.

CHAPTER SEVEN

Diagnosis: Nonepileptic Seizures and Febrile Seizures

37. Patients with refractory seizures sometimes do not have epilepsy.

Many patients (22% in the series by Mattson, 1980) who do not respond to antiepileptic drug therapy do not have epilepsy. They have nonepileptic attacks resembling seizures of epileptic origin but not arising from abnormal neuronal discharge.

If the word 'seizure' is used in its broadest sense to include any paroxysmal attacks with apparent alteration of responsiveness, and/or motor, sensory, or autonomic dysfunction, then it is possible to construct a logical sequence of restrictive terms to describe these phenomena (Table 37.1). Epileptic seizures are most commonly encountered and are, by definition, caused by abnormal neuronal discharge. Other organic seizures involve other systems, such as the cardiovascular system. Metabolic disorders may also be associated with seizures. An overlap between epileptic and other organic seizures is apparent (Desai et al., 1982). Nonorganic seizures are those in which no clear anatomic pathologic change can be correlated with the

Table 37.1.   Some conditions associated with seizures or seizure-like phenomena

Organic conditions	Nonorganic conditions
Epileptic	Psychogenic
Cardiovascular	(hysterical,
aortic stenosis	conversion,
arrhythmias	functional,
vasovagal	pseudoseizures)
orthostatic hypotension	Other psychiatric
Transient cerebral ischemia	disorders (such as
Movement disorders	schizophrenia)
Toxic or metabolic disorders	Sleep disorders
hypoglycemia	Malingering
drug toxicity	
'Headache'	

Modified and expanded from Mattson (1980).

disorder; sleep disorders such as narcolepsy and cataplexy are arbitrarily included in this category.

In 84 patients with nonepileptic seizures studied by Mattson (1980), the most common attacks were associated with hysterical (psychogenic) causes (34 patients), drug toxicity (15 patients), and cerebral ischemia (10 patients). A surprising 75% of the patients improved after appropriate diagnosis and therapy.

38. There is no absolute criterion for psychogenic seizures.

The most frequently encountered of the nonepileptic seizures are psychogenic seizures, also called hysterical or pseudoseizures. The following is exemplary:

> A 12-year-old girl was healthy until she experienced her first seizure at an educational overnight camp. The patient was described as being unresponsive, with her arms and legs shaking. The episode lasted 20 min, but was not associated with incontinence, tongue biting, or postictal abnormality. She had no memory for the attack. An EEG was reported as 'consistent with psychomotor seizures,' and phenytoin was prescribed. During phenytoin therapy, the patient had several witnessed attacks, which began with an interruption of movement and were followed by falling forward or backward, without evident trauma; jerking of all four extremities might then last from a few seconds to a minute. Stevens-Johnson syndrome developed and necessitated hospitalization in an intensive care unit. Phenobarbital was started, but the seizures continued. Carbamazepine and then primidone were added to the regimen, but the attacks continued. The patient was referred for intensive inpatient evaluation of her seizures.
> The results of the neurologic examination and the EEG were normal. Two attacks were recorded; in each attack, the patient gradually fell forward and was unresponsive. She returned quickly to normal consciousness following the attacks, which lasted 10 to 20 sec. No changes were observed in the EEG during the attacks.
> The patient's medications were gradually tapered. She stated spontaneously that she could control all her attacks, and she was discharged, seizure free, on no medication. Follow-up 1 year later revealed no recurrence of seizures.

Psychogenic seizures are more common than has been previously suspected. They also are often difficult to diagnose accurately, and are often mistakenly treated with antiepileptic drugs. Errors of diagnosis and, therefore, of treatment are compounded by the attending physician's erroneous desire to make a hasty diagnosis on the basis of second-hand evidence or even after witnessing an attack. Sometimes it is simply not possible, by observation, to determine the etiology of a seizure, and a considered, rational opinion can be offered only after all data have been collected. According to Desai et al. (1982), the most useful data are provided by simultaneous video and EEG recording of the attacks, recording of the ictal and postictal EEG, and observation of the relationship between antiepileptic medication and seizure frequency (Table 38.1). These three criteria are best applied in a setting of intensive monitoring, which may be the only definitive method of establishing the diagnosis (Desai et al., 1982).

Recorded Attacks

The heterogeneity of psychogenic seizures is limited only by the machinations of the human mind. Epileptic seizures, while varied, have a comparatively limited clinical expression. If the suspected seizure is recorded and compared with epileptic seizures of known etiology, using the International classification of epileptic seizures, a diagnosis of exclusion is often possible. This assumption has three axioms: (1) some patients will have psychogenic attacks that do not resemble either generalized tonic-clonic or complex partial seizures, (2) a certain small but finite group of epileptic seizures will be characterized by unusual events that make classification difficult, and (3) the more experienced the physician in the observation of all types of seizures, the more likely the seizure classification will be correct (Desai et al., 1982).

Ictal and Postical EEG

The EEG is almost always abnormal during an epileptic seizure, especially if consciousness is altered. This observation is helpful in confirming the diagnosis of epilepsy even though many different paroxysmal abnormalities can be observed, especially in partial seizures. Two problems arise in the

Table 38.1 Major criteria: Useful for diagnosing either epileptic or psychogenic seizures

Characteristics	Epileptic seizures		Nonepileptic seizures
	Generalized tonic-clonic seizures	Complex partial seizures	Psychogenic seizures
Comparison of questionable seizure with known seizure types*	Relatively little variation in events	Wide range of events, but most common are well described	Extremely wide range of events with bizarre and unusual behaviour
EEG during seizure	Abnormal and changed from preictal	Almost always abnormal and changed from preictal	Usually normal and unchanged from preictal
EEG immediately after seizure	Almost always abnormal and changed from preictal	Frequently abnormal and changed from preictal	Usually normal and unchanged from preictal
Relation of attacks to medication regimen	Prominent, especially in severely affected patients	Usually related	Usually unrelated

*As described in the international classification of epileptic seizures (Gastaut, 1970).

From Desai et al. (1982).

effective utilization of this criterion. First, in a small percentage of patients with epileptic seizures, the ictal EEG will not show abnormalitites. Second, the ictal EEG is often obscured by movement and muscle artifact, regardless of the etiology of the attack. A good quality recording of the ictal EEG, however, makes a valuable contribution to the diagnosis.

The EEG is almost always abnormal after a generalized tonic-clonic seizure and is frequently abnormal after a complex partial seizure. The postictal EEG has one chief advantage over the ictal EEG: it is less often obscured by artifact, and interpretation of the recording may be easier.

Medication and Seizure Frequency

As Desai et al. (1982) have stated, properly treated epileptic patients show a strong tendency to have fewer seizures when plasma levels of

Table 38.2. Minor criteria: Primarily useful for diagnosing suspected psychogenic seizures

| Characteristics | Epileptic seizures | | Nonepileptic seizures |
	Generalized tonic-clonic seizures	Complex partial seizures	Psychogenic seizures
Onset	Usually paroxysmal, but may be preceded by seizure of different type	Usually paroxysmal, but may be preceded by aura of only a few seconds	Often gradual; prolonged nonspecific warning period may occur
Primary or secondary gain	Rare; a few patients use seizures for secondary gain	Unusual, but a few patients use seizures for secondary gain	Common
Postictal confusion, lethargy, sleepiness	Prominent	Almost always present and often prominent, but may be mild	Often conspicuously absent; patient may be normal immediately after attack
Postictal subjective complaints	Prominent if aroused	Usually prominent; patient rarely feels well	May be smiling or laughing after seizure
Suggestibility	None	Rare	Occasionally
Recollection of events during attack	None	Usually scant and most often none	Sometimes detailed
Violent behavior	None	Rare; virtually always in response to restraint and not highly directed	Rare, though may be highly directed

From Desai et al. (1982).

antiepileptic drugs are adequate. This relationship between medications and seizure regulation can be useful in the assessment of suspected psychogenic seizures. The best procedure is to withdraw medications gradually while the patient is in the hospital and observe for increases in seizure frequency. The likelihood of a correct diagnosis is enhanced by intensive monitoring to record the increased seizure frequency resulting from medication withdrawal.

Numerous other, less important, criteria have been utilized in an attempt to discern which seizures are psychogenic (Table 38.2) and which are epileptic (Table 38.3).

Unfortunately, the positive diagnosis of psychogenic seizures is rarely possible, and *no single criterion should be singled out as diagnostic*. Both psychiatrists and neurologists have attempted to formulate positive criteria for psychogenic seizures — the former by defining the underlying psychiatric

Table 38.3. Minor criteria: Primarily useful for diagnosing suspected epileptic seizures

	Epileptic seizures		Nonepileptic seizures
Characteristics	Generalized tonic-clonic seizures	Complex partial seizures	Psychogenic seizures
Age	Any, past infancy	Any, usually >3yr	Usually older child or adult
Gross tonic-clonic motor phenomena	Always	Rare; seen only in secondarily generalized attacks	None, but resemblance is related to sophistication of mimicry
Tongue biting	Frequent	Rare	Rare
Urinary incontinence	Frequent	Unusual, but not rare	Rare
Abnormal neurologic signs during seizure	May be present	May be present	None
Nocturnal occurrence	Common	May occur	Rare
Injuries sustained as a result of event	Common	Common	Rare, but occasionally occur
Stereotypy of attacks	Relatively little variation	Attacks may or may not be varied, but usually have some consistent patterns	Attacks may or may not be varied; patterns may occasionally be widely divergent

From Desai et al. (1982).

condition and the latter by such tests as changes in serum lactate. The diagnosis, however, remains one of exclusion of other conditions. Also, the separation of hysteria from malingering is often impossible. The coexistence of epileptic and psychogenic seizures in the same patient is not infrequent.

Psychogenic seizures are associated with other types of psychiatric disturbances, in addition to 'hysteria' or 'somatoform disorder.' In fact, depression and schizophrenia are common underlying psychiatric conditions which promote the symptoms of hysteria. Physicians confronted with a patient with apparent psychogenic seizures, therefore, should apply the above criteria and should not be dissuaded by a seemingly inconsistent overall psychiatric diagnosis.

Hyperventilation frequently accompanies psychogenic seizures and is accompanied by tetany as well as dizziness, blurred vision, paresthesias, shortness of breath, and other symptoms (Riley and Roy, 1982). Another group of psychogenic seizures is especially difficult to discern from atonic seizures. Patients, in this group, usually young women, fall without convulsive movements. They may be incontinent of urine, especially if they discover that it will worry their doctors (Walton, 1977).

Finally, patients with psychogenic seizures, even though they may not have epilepsy, are ill and require psychiatric evaluation and care. One approach to therapy is introduction of the concept that the patient can control the attacks. This concept should be introduced slowly, allowing a graceful exit from the psychogenic seizures. Occasionally, the attacks will stop abruptly when the patient is confronted directly; if this technique fails, however, rapport may be lost that might have allowed cessation of the attacks. Therapy of psychogenic seizures is considered in detail in the recent volume by Riley and Roy (1982).

39. Acute anxiety attacks are sometimes mistaken for epileptic seizures.

Increasing recognition of the symptoms of anxiety, coupled with increased incidence of the disorder, has heightened awareness of the acute anxiety attack. The attack itself may take many forms, but the common feature is an overwhelming sense of fear or panic. The fear may be 'free floating' or directed, and although often related to interpersonal encounters, attacks may also occur when the patient is completely alone. Patients are especially vulnerable 'when unaccompanied in the street, in crowds, buses, shops, and particularly when inactive or compelled to wait, as in cinemas or queues' (Harper and Roth, 1962).

Psychophysiologic accompaniments of the attacks include intense sweating, 'spaced-out' or 'detached' feelings, sensations of unreality, palpitations, tachycardia, chest tightness, nausea, vomiting, diarrhea, and dyspnea. Exhaustion may follow an attack. The following is a typical case report:

A 36-year-old woman, an important and fast-rising executive, noticed in late 1977 the onset of 'being detached from the environment,' a feeling which came on suddenly while drinking with her friends. The onset was paroxysmal and disappeared when she was able to go the the bathroom. She had a similar episode a few weeks later and fainted, with loss of consciousness for approximately 20 sec. She had no further alterations of consciousness but began having attacks of panic, with associated feelings of coldness, perspiration, and 'a feeling of detachment,' lasting from half a minute up to many hours, and occurring both at home and at work. A neurologist prescribed phenytoin, which caused her to feel worse, followed by primidone, which made her vomit. She took no medication for 2 months.

The results of the neurologic examination were normal, but the EEG showed left posterior temporal irregular slowing. A diagnosis of acute anxiety attacks was made, and the patient was given diazepam (4 mg/day) as needed for the attacks. She responded dramatically, with striking relief of the severity and frequency of her attacks. A later trial of antidepressant medication was not tolerated. Four years later, she continued to use the diazepam, though usually only once every few months.

The diagnosis of acute anxiety attacks usually rests on three factors. First, the duration of some of the attacks is quite prolonged, up to 15 to 30 min or more — much longer than most epileptic seizures. Second, consciousness is usually not altered during the attack; even though the patient may feel strange, appropriate interaction with the environment is still possible. The patient can almost always recite in detail the events and his or her own actions (unless fainting occurs, as in the patient described above). Hyperventilation may be a prominent feature. Third, the EEG usually does not show epileptiform abnormalities, and the results are often completely normal.

For patients with severe, repetitive episodes of acute anxiety, the chronic use of antidepressants is indicated (Sheehan, 1982). Initial therapy, however, especially in milder cases, may be limited to diazepam, which can be given on either a regular or an as needed basis, often with remarkable effectiveness. Even though no clinical trials have documented its effectiveness, the popularity of diazepam is clearly related to the need to alleviate anxiety in one form or another, and one wonders whether the incidence of acute anxiety is not considerably higher than is reported. The adrenergic hyperactivity can be relieved by the use of propranolol (Easton and Sherman, 1976).

40. Prolonged fugue states are rarely epileptic if highly organized behavior occurs.

Every neurologist is occasionally called upon to consider the possibility of epilepsy in patients who have prolonged attacks (i.e., hours or days) of altered responsiveness to their environment. In most such cases, the medical causes have already been adequately addressed, and the remaining differential diagnosis is between epilepsy and psychiatric disease. More specifically, it is between nonconvulsive status epilepticus (principle 36) and a dissociative disorder. Several kinds of dissociative disorders can be confused with epilepsy. The following descriptions are taken largely from the *Diagnostic and Statistical Manual of Mental Disorders* (American Psychiatric Association, 1980).

Psychogenic amnesia is characterized by a sudden inability to recall important personal information; the disturbance is much more than ordinary forgetfulness. Most commonly, the patient fails to recall all events occurring during a circumscribed period of time.

The patient with *psychogenic fugue* makes a sudden, unexpected trip away from his usual environment; he may assume a new identity and may be confused and disoriented. The patient denies any recollection of the events during the fugue.

The patient with *multiple personalities* has at least two fully integrated personalities that alternately become dominant. Epilepsy is sometimes considered in such patients when the change from one personality to the other is sudden, resembling the paroxysmal onset of a seizure.

Finally, the patient with *depersonalization* has a feeling that the usual sense of one's own reality is temporarily lost or changed; a feeling of unreality pervades the patient's perceptions of his surroundings (principle 22).

The key to the diagnosis can usually be found in a historical analysis of the complexity of the tasks performed during the event. If the patient can barely carry out the tasks of daily living, such as eating and drinking, a continuous seizure state must be considered and evaluated intensively. If, however, the patient disappears from home for two days, then calls home from a distant city and says that he doesn't know what happened or how he got there, then a psychiatric disorder is most likely. A psychiatric diagnosis is especially likely if a number of complicated transactions can be documented during the event, (e.g., changing airplanes, making purchases, arranging accommodations). *The more intricate and complicated the overall performance, the less likely the behavior is to be epileptic.* This fundamental observation also applies to complicated tasks performed during aggressive behavior in which epilepsy is considered in the differential diagnosis (principle 42).

41. Clonic jerking or tonic extension may accompany syncopal episodes.

The neurologist is frequently confronted with a patient who has paroxysmal episodes of alteration of consciousness, with loss of postural tone and clonic jerking and/or tonic extension. In many such patients, the correct diagnosis is not epilepsy but syncope. The following case illustrates the problem:

> A 17-year-old girl was well until the age of 2 years, when she fell and was unresponsive for 1 min; thereafter, she was somewhat 'groggy.' A second, similar episode occurred 4 days later, and although the neurologic examination and EEG showed no abnormalities, she was started on phenobarbital, which she took to the age of 6 years. She had only one further episode, when she was 4 years old.
>
> At 10 years of age, she had loss of consciousness and a few jerking movements at the time of a venipuncture. She then began having attacks several times a year, characterized by loss of consciousness, loss of postural tone, tonic flexion of the arms, and extension of the legs. The attacks lasted 30 to 60 sec and were followed by postictal confusion and headache. They were preceded by dimming of central vision and a feeling of dizziness. She was advised to seek psychiatric care. By the age of 18 years, she was

having one or two attacks a month, and was hospitalized for intensive monitoring because of a sudden increase in attacks to 15 a month. A typical episode was precipitated by venipuncture; dramatic EKG evidence of sinus bradycardia and sinus arrest was documented during the attack.

Syncope is usually defined as an alteration of normal brain function caused by paroxysmal cerebral hypoxia. In most patients, the hypoxia is caused by decreased blood flow to the brain. The various syncopal syndromes have been subdivided into three major and two minor categories by Riley (1982), whose comprehensive list of the etiologies of syncope is found in Table 41.1.

The differential diagnosis of epilepsy and syncope is highly dependent on an adequate medical history. The setting of the attacks may be an important clue to the etiology of the attacks. Some patients, such as the one just described, have stereotyped emotional causes of their attacks; association with venipuncture is common. Many of the same psychologically stressful environments associated with acute anxiety attacks (principle 39) are implicated in syncope as well, and psychogenic attacks, including hyperventilation, must also be considered. Syncope is also precipitated in some patients by

Table 41.1. Syncope

I. Reflex syncopes — vasovagal or vasodepressor syncope
    A. Carotid sinus syndrome
    B. Psychogenic or neurogenic fainting (may be different from 'hysterical' fainting)
    C. Micturition syncope
    D. Tussive syncope
    E. Valsalva-maneuver syncope

II. Syncope due to cardiac causes
    A. Irregularities of rhythm
        1. Heart block with Adams-Stokes syndrome
        2. Supraventricular arrhythmias; sinoatrial block; atrial fibrillation, paroxysmal atrial tachycardia, 'sick sinus syndrome'
        3. Frequent ventricular premature beats
    B. Failure to compensate for sudden drops in peripheral vascular resistance
        1. Congenital heart disease (shunts)
        2. Myxoma
        3. Ball-valve thrombus
        4. Myocardial diseases (myocarditis, degenerative diseases, ischemia)

III. Syncope due to (noncardiac) perfusion failure
    A. Orthostatic hypotension
        1. Hypovolemia
        2. Primary central dysautonomia, CNS degenerative disease (Parkinson's disease)
        3. Autonomic peripheral neuropathy
        4. Medications (mostly antihypertensives)
    B. Shock — may not require postural changes
    C. Cerebrovascular disease

IV. Syncope due to anoxia

V. Syncope with convulsive movements (convulsive syncope)

From Riley and Roy, 1982.

nonanxiety related events, such as micturition and coughing. Patients with syncope often have a prolonged prodrome; the aura in epileptic attacks is usually only a few seconds. Although a few clonic jerks are common in syncope, and tonic extension also occurs, the classic sequence of the generalized tonic-clonic epileptic seizure is rare. The diagnosis can be difficult to establish if the attacks are infrequent. If the spells are frequent or precipitable, monitoring and simultaneous recording of the EEG and EKG is usually definitive. The use of the ambulatory EEG monitor is beneficial when one lead is used to record the EKG (Lai and Ziegler, 1981).

In the 17-year-old girl described above, the vasovagal syncope was unresponsive to cardiac pacing or atropine, demonstrating that bradycardia was not the sole cause of the hypotension. She responded to the use of elastic stockings and leg exercises to minimize the peripheral pooling, which was apparently the result of centrally induced vasodepression (Goldstein et al., 1982).

42. Violence is extremely uncommon during epileptic seizures.

Most epileptiologists agree that violent, aggressive behavior during or after an epileptic seizure occurs almost exclusively in a setting of direct provocation and is more likely to occur in the postictal period.

In an international workshop involving 16 epilepsy centers, 19 epileptic seizures with possible violent behavior were identified from an estimated 5,400 recorded seizures. Eighteen experts from these centers evaluated the 19 attacks by repeated viewing of the video taped seizures. Three attacks were thought to show actual or threatened violence to persons (Delgado-Escueta et al., 1981b). The most severe violent act was an attempt to scratch another persons's face, an act that was typical of the patient's seizures. Depth electrode stimulation of the left hippocampus caused a typical, aggressive seizure (Saint-Hilare et al., 1980). Even this patient could be restrained if held from behind.

The rarity of violence as an ictal event in epileptic patients is supported by the incidence of 0.00019 for unprovoked violence in the highly selected patient population from these referral centers. Such centers specialize in the most difficult and refractory patients.

Although it is admittedly difficult to prove the *non-existence* of ictal violence in epilepsy, conclusions drawn from the above findings can be applied to the vast majority of patients with epilepsy: (1) automatic behavior during seizures is usually brief, fragmentary, and nondirected; most epileptic automatisms are less effective and less directed than normal behavior in the same setting; (2) the more complex and more prolonged the activity, the less likely it is to be epileptic. Complicated acts of violence, therefore, are highly unlikely to be epileptic in origin, and the use of epilepsy as a defense against accusations of violent crime is virtually always unwarranted.

43. Febrile seizures are common and usually benign.

Febrile seizures occur in 2% to 5% of the population (Hauser, 1981). They occur between 3 months and 5 years of age, and are associated with fever, but are not associated with intracranial infection or other defined cause specifically related to the central nervous system. The risk of subsequent epilepsy to most children who experience febrile seizures is minimal and, according to Kendig et al. (1981), therapy generally should be limited to patients with the following risk factors: (1) A family history of nonfebrile seizures, (2) abnormal neurologic or developmental status, and (3) an atypical (prolonged or focal) febrile seizure.

Although there is little evidence that recurrent febrile seizures cause any type of subsequent epilepsy (Fig. 43.1), many physicians prescribe antiepileptic drugs for those patients who have more than two or three febrile seizures, with the object of preventing further, similar attacks. In any case, patients with uncomplicated febrile seizures, even if several eventually occur, are not usually considered to have *epilepsy*, the chronic recurrent disorder. Febrile seizures are self-limiting and usually not associated with any other brain disorder.

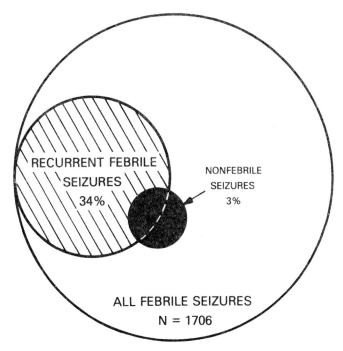

Fig 43.1. In a study of 1,706 children with febrile seizures followed to the age of 7 years (*outer circle*), one-third had recurrent febrile seizures (*hatched circle*). Children with subsequent nonfebrile seizures (epilepsy) came almost equally from among those who did, and those who did not, have at least one recurrence of their febrile seizures. (From Nelson and Ellenberg, 1981.)

44. Continuous, rather than intermittent, therapy is preferred for the prevention of recurrent febrile seizures.

In a collaborative study of 1,706 children with febrile seizures, 1,104 (65%) of them had no further seizures of any type, febrile or nonfebrile, up to the end of the follow-up period at age 7 years (Nelson and Ellenberg, 1976). The treatment of children with a single febrile seizure, without consideration of risk factors, would therefore result in two-thirds of such children receiving drugs for anticipated seizures that would never occur, with or without therapy. If one further considers that even recurrent febrile seizures are not, in themselves, a likely cause of epilepsy, treatment should be limited to the specific subgroups at maximal risk (principle 43).

The reasons for limiting the number of children with febrile seizures who are treated with antiepileptic drugs are related to the difficulties inherent in long-term therapy with powerful remedies. First, the evidence is strong that, in most patients, early recognition of a feverish illness is inadequate and therefore that intermittent therapy is of limited value (Porter, 1981); thus to be effective, therapy must be continuous. Second, continuous therapy is best documented for phenobarbital, a drug with sedating and possible long-term cognitive effects. The continuous use of valproate may be effective, but idiosyncratic hepatotoxicity limits its usefulness, especially for a relatively benign disorder such as febrile seizures. No other nonsedative drugs appear to be effective in stopping recurrences. Third, even continuous therapy requires attention to the underlying assumptions that (1) a steady state drug level can be established and maintained, (2) the steady state level is effective (i.e., therapeutic), (3) parents or guardians can and will continue to administer the drug as prescribed, (4) associated illness or therapy for such illness will not interfere with drug efficacy (Porter, 1981).

Evidence suggests that a plasma phenobarbital level of approximately 15 μg/ml is sufficient for preventing the recurrence of febrile seizures in most patients (Porter, 1981). The difficulty in giving phenobarbital, or probably any other medication, continuously is summarized well by Wolf (1981), who reported that 'even in a selected group of parents concerned enough to be willing to participate in a research study, compliance in a significant majority is achieved only by considerable exhortation, follow-up, and monitoring by the physician. Many parents are very, very reluctant to give their apparently well child a drug day after day.'

Finally, the above discussion relates solely to the prevention of *recurrent febrile seizures* and not to the prevention of epilepsy. Treatment of recurrent (or complex) febrile seizures to prevent epilepsy remains a speculative therapeutic approach. On the other hand, epileptic patients with nonfebrile seizures should obviously be treated for their epilepsy, regardless of whether they do or do not have febrile seizures.

CHAPTER EIGHT

Therapy: General Considerations

45. Be certain that the patient has epilepsy before prescribing antiepileptic drugs.

Antiepileptic drugs are primarily useful for the treatment of recurrent abnormal neuronal discharges — epilepsy. Other conditions, such as bipolar depression, myotonia, and trigeminal neuralgia, may also be treated with certain antiepileptic drugs; Klawans (1979) has summarized several such uses. Unfortunately, since many patients with well-documented epilepsy continue to have seizures, physicians become inured to the many patients who, though their seizures are properly diagnosed and properly treated, simply do not get better. True though this may be for many patients with intractable seizures, the resulting attitude of hopelessness causes a failure to recognize that some patients who fail to respond to treatment have either the wrong diagnosis or the wrong therapy.

Epilepsy should virtually always be a positive diagnosis; when the diagnosis is uncertain, a therapeutic trial of antiepileptic drugs is rarely successful. When psychogenic seizures are incorrectly diagnosed as epilepsy, for example, administration of antiepileptic drugs may result in a temporary placebo effect, temporary worsening of the condition, or intolerance to the medication. Eventually, confusion reigns as more drugs at higher doses are tried. The chief pitfalls in the diagnosis of epilepsy include not only psychogenic seizures (principle 38) but also acute anxiety attacks (principle 39), dissociative states (principle 40), and syncope (principle 41).

Numerous studies have shown that a single drug controls seizures in many patients and that 'polytherapy' is often unnecessary. Patients always deserve at least one trial of monotherapy; a different drug can be tried if the first is unsuccessful. Refractory epilepsy, however, will usually be better controlled with more than one drug (Porter et al., 1980).

One area of particular concern to pediatricians is the proper diagnosis of 'abdominal epilepsy.' The epigastric aura (with or without a 'rising sensation') is the most common premonitory symptom in complex partial seizures, and abdominal symptoms also occur in children with seizures. Vomiting and abdominal pain may occur in association with altered responsiveness, other signs of epilepsy, and abnormal EEG findings. The onset of the attacks is usually paroxysmal, and postictal sleepiness is the rule. Although the diagnosis is frequently considered, especially in children who have recurrent episodes of abdominal pain and vomiting, 'only a small proportion of these children have abdominal epilepsy' (Menkes, 1980), even if a gastrointestinal evaluation is unrevealing. The diagnosis should not be made on the basis of the abdominal symptoms alone, but on the positive criteria noted above. Childhood migraine should especially be considered in the differential diagnosis.

46. The seizure diagnosis determines the appropriate therapy.

The kind of seizures that a patient has determines the correct medication or other therapy. This highly empirical approach still predominates in spite of continuing efforts to establish more basic and more rational diagnostic methods. The likelihood that basic neuroscience will contribute to the precise diagnosis of epilepsy still seems many years away. We do know, however, that the antiepileptic drugs now available are often considerably specific for various types of epileptic seizures and that proper seizure classification (principle 14) is crucial to appropriate therapy.

The clinical evidence for specificity against various seizure types is impressive. Consider the following information:

1. Some drugs, such as phenytoin or carbamazepine, are virtually ineffective against absence seizures or myoclonic seizures, but control partial seizures and most generalized tonic-clonic seizures.
2. Some drugs, such as ethosuximide or trimethadione, have no effect against partial seizures, generalized tonic-clonic seizures, or myoclonic seizures, but are useful in treating absence seizures.
3. Valproate is effective against both absence seizures and myoclonic seizures, but is less effective against other kinds of attacks. The drug may, however, be effective against generalized tonic-clonic seizures.
4. Phenytoin is useful against most generalized tonic- clonic attacks, but is often ineffective for alcohol withdrawal seizures (unlike, for example, barbiturates).
5. Corticotropin (ACTH) may stop infantile spasms, but has little effect on other seizure types.

Although the basic mechanism of each of the seizure types is presumably related to the different response to various drugs, we still have only primitive notions about these seizure mechanisms and about how antiepileptic drugs act to prevent their occurrence. Experimental data suggest that the variability of the various seizure types and their differential response to medication is complex. As we are likely to continue with empirical rather than rational therapy for a considerable time to come, the refinement of empirical approaches has a legitimate role for both practitioners and clinical investigators.

47. Frequently reevaluate the patient with intractable seizures.

Together, the diagnostic and therapeutic principles in this book recommend a vigorous effort on the part of both the physician and the patient to improve seizure control and reduce medication toxicity. This effort often cannot be accomplished quickly. It cannot be accomplished at all without frequent reevaluation and medication adjustments. The following summary, quoted from an actual neurologic consultation, illustrates the problem:

> This 12-year-old girl has had identical episodes of loss of consciousness associated with body stiffness preceded by frontal headaches since the age of two, with the last two attacks occurring two weeks ago while on no anticonvulsive medication. A recent EEG as well as two previous EEG's were all within normal limits. Neurological examination negative....Impression — seizure disorder R/O syncopal attacks....Comment — the lack of precipitating factors and the early onset would be against syncope. However, it remains to be proven either clinically or electroencephalographically that the patient suffers from epilepsy. I advised the mother should the patient have another attack to check the patient's pulse....In the meantime, we should assume that the patient suffers from epileptic seizures and treat her appropriately. I chose Mysoline [primidone]...I gave instructions so that the patient will start taking 50 mg twice a day and gradually will increase to 250 mg twice a day. *I plan to see [the child] in one year* [italics mine].

The proposed 1-year follow-up of this child precludes any meaningful possibility of establishing the correct diagnosis in a reasonable time period. As it turns out, the child did not have epilepsy. The correct diagnosis was needlessly delayed. Even if the diagnosis had been correct, the plan to start medication with a gradually increasing dosage, without monitoring, meant that adverse reactions might go unnoticed and that the dosage was merely assumed to be efficacious. Finally, this example typifies some of the difficulties of therapeutic drug trials to establish the correct diagnosis.

48. The role of psychologic methods in the treatment of the epilepsies remains limited.

The use of psychologic methods in the treatment of epilepsy is difficult to evaluate. Their most promising application is to the reflex epilepsies, which may be refractory to standard antiepileptic therapies and may respond to deconditioning. Such patients have a specific triggering factor in their seizures, and various psychologic techniques may be used to decrease the sensitivity of the patient to the stimulus (Forster and Booker, 1975). Typical stimuli include bright or flashing light, visual patterns, reading, eating, speaking, or listening to music. The benefits of psychologic therapy are unquestionably excellent in many cases of reflex epilepsy.

The reflex epilepsies, however, represent only a small subset of the total population of epileptic patients. Hence attempts have been made to introduce conditioning techniques, such as biofeedback, to epileptic patients with other types of seizures or to subgroups whose seizures appear to be triggered by stress. Many problems arise in evaluating data from studies designed to demonstrate the efficacy of such methods. First, environmental changes affect seizure frequency (Riley et al., 1981), and the studies must control these variables. The seizure frequency may be decreased, for example, simply by increasing the attention paid to the patient by physicians, nurses, or other interested professionals. Second, the group of patients treated by psychologic methods may not be homogeneous with regard to the seizure diagnosis (principle 14), thereby making evaluation of the group data difficult or impossible.

In summary, because highly motivated and well-meaning investigators of psychologic methods of treatment may inadvertently convey their enthusiasm to the study patients, there is a need for rigorous controls of both the study design and the population studied. Currently, psychologic methods should be limited to the treatment of the few patients in whom specific deconditioning is possible or to well-controlled investigations on carefully defined subgroups of patients.

CHAPTER NINE

Therapy: Pharmacology and Pharmacokinetics

49. Give drugs after meals and at bedtime to maximize total daily intake without toxicity.

Multiple daily doses are important for drugs with short half-lives and/or gastrointestinal toxicity. When the drug has a short half-life (principle 50), frequent administration during the day will reduce peaks and troughs in its plasma level. If the drug is administered after meals, the absorption rate will be retarded, and the smoothing effect on the plasma drug level will be enhanced. When mixed with food, the drug gradually enters the bloodstream, avoiding a peak plasma drug level which can cause toxicity. In addition, patients usually tolerate bedtime doses quite well, unless they get up after retiring for the night.

The administration of drugs after meals and at bedtime is especially effective for patients requiring maximal antiepileptic drug doses for seizure control. Taking the drug after meals also ameliorates direct gastric irritation, regardless of whether the drug has a short half-life (e.g., valproate) or a long half-life (e.g., ethosuximide). For example, many patients who routinely omit breakfast have gastric distress from the morning drug dose. This local effect may be important for patients who have a sensitive gastrointestinal tract even though they require only a moderate amount of drug for seizure control.

Some drugs can be administered infrequently and with little attention to the time of day or relation to meals. The most publicized of these antiepileptic drugs is phenytoin, in which once-a-day administration has become popular. Some patients find such a regimen convenient and entirely satisfactory, but others are bothered by toxic effects and find that twice-a-day administration eliminates unpleasant side effects. More importantly, some generic phenytoin preparations are more rapidly absorbed than proprietary formulations. The rapidly absorbed preparations (called 'prompt release') are even more likely to cause toxicity on a once-a-day regimen, and package inserts may specifically contraindicate a single daily dose. (Food and Drug Administration, 1981).

50. The key to drug intake intervals is the drug's half-life.

The spacing of antiepileptic drugs throughout the day should not be based on intuition and instinct: more effective and more scientific methods are available. From a pharmacokinetic standpoint, it makes no difference whether long half-life drugs are given frequently or infrequently. If maximum therapeutic effectiveness of the short half-life drugs is desired, however, they must be delivered frequently — often four times a day. The rule is simple: give short half-life drugs frequently. If the importance of this regimen (principle 49) is carefully explained, most patients will adhere to it.

The principle behind this recommendation is that short half-life drugs are cleared from the body faster than long half-life drugs. Indeed, the time a drug takes to decline to half its previous (arbitrary) level in the blood is defined as its half-life. For example, a drug which at noon has a plasma level of 20 µg/ml and at 6 p.m. has a level of 10 µg/ml (assuming no drug intake during the interval) has a half-life of 6 hr, which is a rather short half-life for an antiepileptic drug.

Two antiepileptic drugs, valproate and carbamazepine, have short half-lives. When valproate is given only every 12 hr, its plasma level fluctuates widely (Fig. 50.1). It is most important, therefore, to space out the administration of these drugs during the day, especially in patients whose

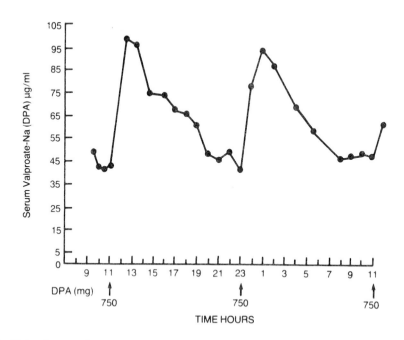

Fig. 50.1. Serum valproate fluctuations in a 12-hr dosing schedule. (Modified from Rowan et al., 1979.)

attacks are not completely controlled and who require maximum effectiveness from the limited antiepileptic armamentarium. The same recommendation applies to a lesser extent to primidone, whose antiepileptic action is complicated by its long half-life metabolite, phenobarbital.

51. The key to intervals between changes in drug dose is the drug's half-life.

The disadvantage of drugs with short half-lives is the necessity of frequent administration (principle 50). The advantage of drugs with short half-lives is the ability to change from one steady-state level to another in a relatively short time. The pharmacokinetic rule is simple: after every dose change it takes five half-lives to reach 97% of a new steady-state plasma drug level. Only after the new steady-state level is reached can drug efficacy be evaluated. For example, accurate evaluation of the efficacy of phenobarbital within a few days after a dose change is not possible. The half-life of phenobarbital may be 96 hr or more, and 3 weeks will often be required to reach a new steady-state level. With carbamazepine or valproate, however, a new steady state will be achieved within a few days, and the efficacy of the drug can be more rapidly determined. Of the antiepileptic drugs most commonly used, only carbamazepine and valproate, and to some extent primidone, have short half-lives, which allow relatively rapid achievement of a steady-state level after a dose change (Table 51.1).

This principle emphasizes the need to wait for the achievement of the steady-state plasma drug level prior to evaluation of the drug's efficacy at the new level. The same emphasis also applies to dose-related toxicity. Dose-related toxicity, like efficacy, cannot be fully evaluated until the new steady-state level is achieved. Because a patient tolerates a 400-mg daily dose of phenytoin for the first 3 days of administration does not mean that toxicity will not occur after 1 week at that dose (principle 64).

Occasionally, toxicity occurs before a steady-state level is reached, and a

Table 51.1 Plasma half-life of six antiepileptic drugs

Drug	Half-life	Time to reach steady state
Carbamazepine	12 hr	3 days
Valproate	12 hr	3 days
Primidone*	12 hr	3 days
Phenytoin	1 day	5 days**
Ethosuximide	2 days	10 days
Phenobarbital	4 days	3 weeks

*Primidone is converted rapidly to phenobarbital (principle 87).
**Phenytoin obeys saturation kinetics (principle 64).
Modified from Penry and Newmark, 1979.

dosage decrease is indicated. Seizure control theoretically could also be evaluated before a steady-state level is attained, allowing for a lower dosage, but efficacy is best evaluated after steady state is achieved.

Seizure frequency will also affect the time required for efficacy evaluation. If a patient is having five seizures a day, for example, the efficacy can be determined quickly. If the patient is having only two seizures a year, a long time will be required to see whether the regimen is satisfactory.

52. The time needed to reach a steady-state plasma drug level is not determined by the amount of the dose change.

Whether the dose of an antiepileptic drug is increased by 15 mg or by 150 mg daily, the time necessary to achieve a new steady-state level is the same. Although this assumption is based on linear kinetics, only phenytoin has deviated from this model (principle 64). Explained another way, the eventual *height* of the new steady-state plasma drug level is a function of the daily dose of the drug, whereas the *time* needed to reach this steady-state level is related not to the total dose nor to the amount of the dose change but to the half-life of the drug (Fig. 52.1). The longer the half-life, the longer the time needed to reach steady state, regardless of the dose or the amount of dose change.

One way to avoid the long time needed to reach a steady-state level when using long half-life drugs is to load the patient with an initial large dose. This procedure is most useful with phenytoin (principle 85) and least practical, but still possible, with barbiturates or benzodiazepines.

When changing the dose of a drug, especially at higher plasma levels,

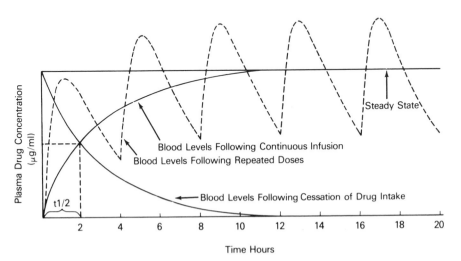

Fig. 52.1. Fluctuation of plasma drug levels with repeated drug administration (*dotted lines*). The steady state level after five to seven half-lives approaches that achieved by continuous infusion. In this case, the half-life of the drug is only 2 hr. (From Porter, 1981.)

changes should be made slowly and in small increments. Dose-related toxicity, when encountered, will thereby be relatively mild.

53. Use the therapeutic plasma drug level only as a guide.

Many tables of optimal therapeutic plasma drug levels for various antiepileptic drugs have been published; a simplified version is found in Table 53.1. The usual therapeutic level of phenytoin, for example, is 10 to 20 μg/ml, which suggests that most patients will experience optimal seizure control with minimal toxicity if their plasma phenytoin level is within this range. Unfortunately, there are many exceptions to this guideline, and many patients are well controlled at higher or lower levels. For example, as illustrated by the following case report, some patients tolerate phenytoin levels exceeding 20 μg/ml and require these high levels for seizure control:

A 17-year-old boy had a 7-year history of complex partial and generalized tonic-clonic seizures; the seizures occurred almost daily. The EEG showed bilateral epileptiform abnormalities. The patient tolerated a 400-mg daily dose of phenytoin, with plasma phenytoin levels near 15 μg/ml, but the seizures remained uncontrolled. Phenytoin was gradually increased to 550 mg/day, at which time the patient became seizure free; he had minimal nystagmus, but no diplopia or ataxia. He continued to be seizure free for several years on this dose, which gave plasma phenytoin levels of 35 to 45 μg/ml. An attempt to decrease the dose was unsuccessful. When a plasma phenytoin level of 25 μg/ml was attained with dose reduction, complex partial seizures recurred and the patient asked to be given the higher dose, even though the potential toxicity of phenytoin was explained to him. He again become seizure free on the higher dose.

In consideration of the lower dose of phenytoin that may be effective in seizure control, it is noteworthy that a 300-mg daily dose of phenytoin, the 'usual' neurologic dose, half the time gives a plasma phenytoin level of less than 10 μg/ml (Porter and Layzer, 1975), but which appears to give adequate seizure control in some patients. The concept of seizure control and its relation

Table 53.1. Effective plasma levels of six antiepileptic drugs

Drug	Effective level (μg/ml)	High effective level* (μg/ml)	Toxic level (μg/ml)
Carbamazepine	4-10	7	>8
Primidone	5-15	10	>12
Phenytoin	10-20	18	>20
Phenobarbital	10-40	35	>40
Ethosuximide	50-100	80	>100
Valproate	50-100	80	>100

*Level that should be achieved, if possible, in patients with refractory seizures, assuming that the blood samples are drawn before administration of the morning medication (principle 58).

to plasma phenytoin levels has been reviewed by Kutt (1982).

The main considerations in the use of plasma drug levels are as follows (Porter, 1983a):

1. Antiepileptic drug monitoring is used only as a guide to changes in therapy; it is not a substitute for clinical judgment.
2. Expected therapeutic plasma drug levels are average values; each patient will have an individually optimal value.
3. The determinations help achieve maximal effects of each medication. The use of gradually increasing doses to establish the maximally tolerated dose is a valid concept in patients with refractory seizures.
4. The determinations are invaluable in the presence of toxic side effects, especially in patients taking multiple drugs.
5. Noncompliance, malabsorption, and altered metabolism can be identified, but only noncompliance is a common problem (principle 56).
6. A reliable laboratory is critical to proper interpretation of the results (principle 55). If the blood samples for determination of plasma drug levels are drawn at various times during the day, such levels may be misleading (principle 54).

54. Monitor the plasma drug level first thing in the morning.

One of the most confusing aspects of monitoring plasma levels of antiepileptic drugs arises because determinations are made on blood samples obtained randomly at various times during the day. Unfortunately, data from such determinations are occasionally used to support the argument that a dose-to-plasma level relationship does not exist for a particular drug. Especially with short half-life drugs, it is important to establish a fixed relationship between drug intake and blood sampling. Since it is virtually impossible to obtain blood samples during the day under controlled conditions, the only rational time to take routine samples is in the morning, before the first dose of medication is administered. Such samples reflect the base-line (trough) level and are directly comparable. Changes in doses can thereby be confidently followed by monitoring plasma drug levels, without fear of artifactual effects from the numerous variables (e.g., influence of food on rate of absorption, time of venipuncture). Inconvenience to the patient is often considerable, but the data are well worth the effort, especially in difficult cases. If the epilepsy clinic is held in the morning, rather than in the afternoon, patients can delay taking their morning dose until after the blood sample is obtained.

To detect the toxic offender in a multidrug regimen, it is sometimes better to take blood samples at times other than in the morning. This is rarely necessary, however, because the levels determined from the morning samples will usually indicate which drug is present in the blood at a high level.

55. A reliable clinical laboratory is critical for accurate monitoring of plasma drug levels.

If there is one area where antiepileptic treatment is in the forefront of the therapeutics of chronic disease, it is in the use of plasma drug level determinations as a guide to therapy. Unfortunately, the quality of the determinations varies considerably from laboratory to laboratory. This poor performance was documented in a blind survey of clinical laboratories (Pippenger et al., 1976). Half the laboratory determinations reported were outside one standard deviation of those obtained on the same samples in five reference laboratories and were erroneous to a degree that would mislead the doctor. This is especially disturbing to those who are attempting to convince physicians of the value of these levels and to encourage their use.

It is incumbent upon each physician to be certain that the laboratory he uses is competent (i.e., the reported values are near to the correct or true values) and reliable (i.e., the laboratory consistently gives accurate results). The laboratory should subscribe to a quality control program. Two such programs are available in the United States. Information on these programs can be obtained from the American Association of Clinical Chemistry, 1725 K Street N.W., Washington, D.C. 20006 U.S.A., or from the College of American Pathologists, 7400 N. Skokie Blvd., Skokie, Illinois 60076 U.S.A. These programs are not expensive to join and have had a positive effect on the average quality of antiepileptic drug determinations. For example, when the poorly performing laboratories mentioned above were reevaluated, 88% were performing satisfactorily, based on monthly proficiency samples (Pippenger et al., 1977). If a clinical laboratory is not willing to join a quality control program, or if it is not willing to share the results of its determinations on unknown samples, the physician should be concerned about the results he receives from that laboratory.

Some of the common laboratory errors are often related to inadequate standard reference material. Such errors include the inadequate use of primary standards of different concentrations to cover a range of determined values (Kupferberg and Penry, 1975), but the availability of reliable reference standards is equally important. To obtain highly accurate determinations of antiepileptic drugs, a standard reference material in a biologic matrix is required (Kupferberg and Penry, 1975). These highly precise standard reference materials have now been developed by the U.S. National Bureau of Standards for carbamazepine, ethosuximide, phenobarbital, phenytoin, primidone, and valproate. Three standards for each drug are available, with concentrations in the subtherapeutic, therapeutic, and toxic ranges. Inquiries regarding the availability of these standards should be sent to Office of Standard Reference Materials, Room B311, Chemistry Building, National Bureau of Standards, Washington D.C. 20234 U.S.A.

56. Noncompliance is the principal cause of uncontrolled seizures.

Poor compliance with the physician's instructions regarding medication is not a problem unique to epilepsy; it is a difficulty encountered in the therapy of any chronic disease for which daily therapy is indicated. The typical patient with infrequent seizures forgets for a myriad of reasons to take his medications and continues to have seizures. The frustrated doctor prescribes higher and higher doses of drugs, observing neither toxic effects nor seizure control. Then, if the patient suddenly becomes compliant, toxicity occurs swiftly; the doctor is dumbfounded and the patient disillusioned. It is an even more difficult problem if the patient has intractable seizures or deliberately omits medication (Fig. 56.1). Poor compliance is by no means limited to patients of lower socioeconomic backgrounds. Children from socioeconomically advantaged families, for example, may resist compliance in spite of logical explanations and emotional cajoling. Sometimes such forgetfulness can be detected by the pattern of the plasma drug levels (Fig. 56.2).

There are several ways of improving compliance. Even with complicated regimens, compliance is indeed possible if the patient is capable of learning:

1. For patients who seem apathetic about their problems, emphasize the importance of taking the prescribed doses so that the physician can interpret the results of therapy.

2. Be understanding and forgiving but firm with patients who are capable of good compliance. At the first visit, it may be useful to reach an understanding of the importance of regular drug intake. Compliance is a reasonable price to pay for improved seizure control, and the physician should expect it.

3. Ask about drug compliance frequently. Have the patient (or guardian who manages the pills) recite, at each visit, the number of each tablet taken and when each is taken during the day. The patient will come to expect the question and will therefore learn the daily regimen. Since alternate day regimens (e.g., 300 and 400 mg of phenytoin on alternate days) are unnecessary and a good excuse for getting confused, they should not be used (instead, for example, give 350 mg/day of phenytoin).

4. An effective technique for improving compliance, and one that the physician should insist on in difficult cases, is the 'morning set-up' plan. Insist that the patient (or guardian) count out the entire day's dose of medications on awakening in the morning; place the tablets in a designated place such as a cup or separate pillbox. Draw from this receptacle as needed for the day's dose and inspect it at bedtime to be sure that the day's dose is entirely consumed. Repeat the procedure each day. Well-educated patients will resist such an elementary procedure; ignore these complaints and insist that it be followed.

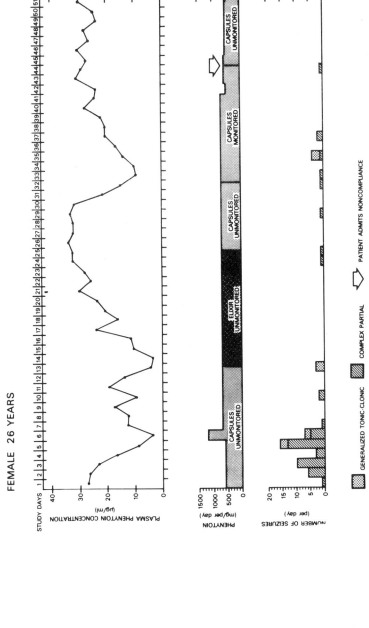

Fig. 56.1. Graphic representation of plasma phenytoin concentrations and phenytoin dosage in relation to number of seizures in a hospitalized 26-year-old woman with deliberate non-compliance. During days 1 through 13, she had many seizures and erratic levels; capsules were unmonitored. During days 14 through 25, she was given phenytoin elixir; plasma drug levels rose and seizure control improved dramatically. On day 26 she was again started on phenytoin capsules unmonitored; the levels fell and seizures recurred. On day 33, the patient's mouth was inspected with each (daily) phenytoin dose. The levels again rose and seizures abated. On day 45, she admitted throwing the medicine into the commode. She was discharged with excellent seizure control, but 1 year later we received a long-distance phone call from a physician with a fascinating patient (the same) who could not absorb phenytoin! (From Desai et al., 1978.)

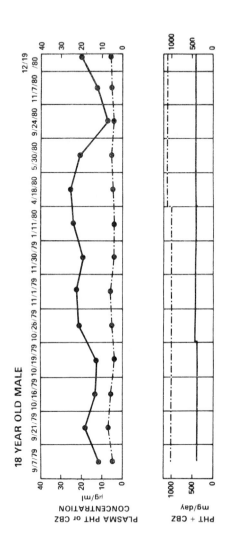

Fig. 56.2. The 18-year-old son of a prominent scientist had gradually increasing doses and plasma levels of phenytoin (*solid line*) and carbamazepine (*dotted line*), which correlated with improved control of his complex partial seizures until he left home for college in September 1980. On September 19 and 20, he had several secondarily generalized tonic-clonic seizures in the college dormitory. He was taken home on September 21, and blood drug levels were determined 3 days later on September 24. The phenytoin (PHT) level had fallen dramatically from the level in May 1980, but the carbamazepine (CBZ) was apparently unchanged. This puzzling observation was explained by the parents' careful monitoring of drug intake during the patient's 3 days at home. Carbamazepine, with a short half-life, returned quickly to a steady state, and by September 24, the level was again therapeutic. Phenytoin, however, with a relatively long half-life, took much longer to return to steady state, and the September 24 level was therefore low. Seizure control returned after drug intake was resumed.

CHAPTER TEN

Therapy: Partial Seizures

57. Use carbamazepine or phenytoin for partial seizures.

Partial seizures respond to carbamazepine, hydantoins, and barbiturates. The drugs of choice, however, are the first two, and choosing between them is usually related to factors other than efficacy. Phenytoin and carbamazepine are approximately equally effective; this has been recognized in Europe for many years, but only rather recently in the United States.

The choice of phenytoin as the primary drug has several advantages. It is an old, safe compound, and most physicians are familiar with its use. Serious side effects are rare and almost always reversible. Plasma phenytoin level determinations are commonly available, and dose-related toxicity is rarely a serious problem (principle 66). Disadvantages of phenytoin use include hirsutism, gingival hyperplasia, coarsening of the features, and a teratogenic potential, including the fetal hydantoin syndrome (principle 93). Phenytoin was discovered in the late 1930's, and was marketed before controlled clinical trials were required. Its effectiveness against partial seizures and generalized tonic-clonic seizures is documented, if only anecdotally.

The choice of carbamazepine has several advantages. It is easily tolerated by most patients, does not cause hirsutism or gingival hyperplasia, and may have a positive psychotropic effect. Disadvantages of carbamazepine use include the risk of blood dyscrasias (an overrated fear), and its short half-life, which may require a dosing schedule of several times a day. Carbamazepine was first used as an antiepileptic drug in the early 1960's (Penry and Porter, 1979), at which time it was reported in Europe to be an effective agent. Later, two trials were reported in the United States. Rodin et al. (1974) conducted a double-blind study of carbamazepine added to phenytoin and phenobarbital in 37 patients. Carbamazepine reduced the frequency of complex partial seizures by 83% and generalized tonic-clonic seizures by 55%. Cereghino et al. (1974) evaluated carbamazepine in a complex study design in which three groups of patients received phenytoin, phenobarbital, or carbamazepine. Carbamazepine was shown to be as effective as the other two drugs in preventing partial and generalized tonic-clonic seizures.

Most important, neither phenytoin nor carbamazepine sedates the patient. It is for this reason that barbiturates are second line drugs against partial seizures.

58. Plasma drug levels should be at the upper end of the therapeutic range in patients with refractory epilepsy.

The optimal drug level for any individual patient is the level that controls the seizures without toxic side effects. In patients with refractory epilepsy, in which more than one drug is employed, one usually needs to be certain that all drugs are at maximally tolerated doses. Monitoring of plasma drug levels can be critical in determining which doses should be increased or decreased to achieve maximal seizure control with minimal toxicity. The following case report is exemplary:

A 20-year-old man had the onset of generalized tonic-clonic seizures at the age of 8 years, followed by complex partial seizures at the age of 9 years. The latter were characterized by a simple partial onset, with 'ringing in the ears,' followed by staring, drooling, and loss of consciousness for 2 min, followed by a gradual return to normal consciousness over 3 to 5 min. Tiredness followed each attack. By age 16 years, the patient was having monthly seizures, and his behavior at home was nearly intolerable; it was clearly worsened by barbiturates. A regimen of phenytoin and carbamazepine was started. Although these two drugs had previously been tried, the maximally tolerated dose of phenytoin had been 300 mg/day, and carbamazepine 800 mg/day. Over many months, the barbiturate was discontinued, and phenytoin and carbamazepine were increased, using a four-times-a-day regimen (similar to that described in principle 60). Each drug was pushed to maximally tolerated doses, with occasional temporary toxicity from each. Diplopia was the presenting sign of toxicity for each drug, and plasma drug levels were measured to determine which drug was the toxic offender. Eventually, the patient was able to tolerate 425 mg/day of phenytoin and 1,100 mg/day of carbamazepine. From morning blood samples, plasma levels of phenytoin remained in the range of 17 to 20 μg/ml, and plasma levels of carbamazepine in the range of 6.5 to 7.5 μg/ml.

On this regimen, the patient's behavior improved dramatically, and his seizures decreased from one a month to one every 6 months. He graduated from high school, and is in his third year of college.

The approach to patients with seizures that are difficult to control is fundamentally the same as before the advent of monitoring plasma drug levels. The object is to maximize the effect of efficacious antiepileptic drugs without producing unacceptable toxic effects. In patients whose seizures are controlled without dose increases or changing to other drugs, no problem exists. In difficult patients, however, the therapeutic range of plasma drug levels should be considered only a rough guide to the patient's tolerance. The 'push to toxicity' approach is most valid, of course, for nonsedative drugs, since dose-related side effects of phenytoin and carbamazepine have a relatively sharp onset at certain levels, depending on the individual patient. Phenobarbital, on the other hand, causes slight sedation at low levels (principle 86) which very gradually worsens with higher levels. When extraordinary levels of 70 to 90 μg/ml are attained, the patient may still be ambulatory and seemingly unconcerned, and, to the insensitive, may appear to be tolerating the drug well.

Monitoring of plasma drug levels is invaluable in the process of achieving maximal effect of more than one drug simultaneously. When using a combination of phenytoin and carbamazepine in a patient with intractable complex partial seizures, for example, it is possible, as the upper range of both drugs is approached, to tell which of the two is actually causing toxic side effects by measuring plasma levels of each drug simultaneously. The maximally tolerated plasma drug levels for most patients — the levels the physician should aim for in difficult patients — are listed in Table 53.1.

59. A 1000-mg daily dose of carbamazepine is often not enough for an adult.

In adults whose seizures are difficult to control, and for which carbamazepine is appropriate, a 1,000-mg daily dose of carbamazepine is usually insufficient to achieve maximal benefit of the drug. The reason that many doctors do not prescribe higher doses is twofold: (1) the drug has a reputation, especially in the United States, for causing severe hematologic side effects, and (2) inadequate attention is given to the regimen, causing the occurrence of dose-related side effects at low and suboptimal total daily doses. Resolution of these two problems allows patients to benefit from higher doses; idiosyncratic side effects are considered in principle 67, and dose-related side effects in principle 65.

Monitoring the plasma carbamazepine level can be useful in obtaining the maximal effect from the drug. In most, though by no means all, adults, 1,000 mg/day will give a morning level of only about 4 to 5 μg/ml. Most patients can tolerate a morning level of at least 6.5 to 7 μg/ml, recognizing that the level will be somewhat higher at various times during the day. To achieve such levels, doses of 1,200 to 1,400 mg/day are common, and some patients tolerate 2,000 mg/day without symptoms of toxicity. Only the elderly, who may not tolerate doses of more than 400 to 600 mg/day, and those whose seizures are well controlled on lower doses, should not be tried on relatively high doses of carbamazepine.

60. Increase the carbamazepine dose in 100-mg increments after a 1,000-mg daily dose has been achieved.

Carbamazepine does not obey saturation kinetics, as does phenytoin, but the approach to using higher doses is much the same. Another difference between phenytoin and carbamazepine is the relatively short half-life of the latter, which allows more rapid dose changes. It is useful, nevertheless, to approach dose-related toxicity slowly. This means increasing the dose in 100-mg increments in adults. Such changes should not be made more often than every 3 or 4 days, and at higher levels it is useful to wait 2 or 3 weeks between changes. The appearance of toxicity at a particular time of the day may require rearrangement of the dose, often without decreasing the total daily dose; such rearrangement is especially useful if the toxicity is mild.

A typical patient with complex partial seizures is on the following regimen:

	Phenytoin	Carbamazepine
After breakfast	150 mg	300 mg
After lunch		400 mg
After dinner		300 mg
Bedtime	200 mg	300 mg
Total daily dose	350 mg	1,300 mg

If the patient complains of 30 min of double vision at 1 or 2 p.m., make certain that he is taking his drugs *after* lunch, and, if so, consider moving 100 mg of carbamazepine from after lunch to bedtime, leaving the total daily dose unchanged.

The above regimen is more complicated than is usually prescribed. The patient is required to take two sizes of phenytoin (50 mg and 100 mg) and two sizes of carbamazepine (100 mg and 200 mg), and has a four-times-a-day dosing schedule. Patients with difficult seizure problems will adapt to such a schedule if it is mandated to them from the beginning and if the doctor is both convinced of its importance and persistent in his efforts to enforce compliance.

Finally, carbamazepine may induce its own metabolism, and the optimal steady-state concentration at the maximally tolerated dose may not be attainable until 10 to 14 days after introduction of the drug.

61. A 300-mg daily dose of phenytoin is often not enough for an adult.

Incremental increases in phenytoin unfortunately have been related to the size of the most commonly used capsule, that is, 100 mg. The 'standard' adult dose of phenytoin is 300 mg/day, and many physicians are reluctant to prescribe higher doses. This reluctance is reinforced by the correct observation that 400 mg/day, the next increment usually attempted, causes toxicity in a considerable number of patients. The often erroneous conclusion is that 300 mg/day is all that the patient can tolerate. Several studies have shown that 300 mg/day in most adults yields plasma phenytoin levels of only 8 to 12 μg/ml, which are often below the therapeutic range and certainly not near the maximally tolerated level. To obtain maximal benefit from this valuable drug, the dose must be increased in small increments at doses exceeding 300 mg/day (principle 62), with careful attention to saturation kinetics (principle 64).

Although high plasma levels of phenytoin have been reported to cause seizures, several studies have been unable to document that such increases in seizure frequency are common, especially in the absence of overt toxicity (Bazemore and Zuckermann, 1974; Porter et al., 1980). Exacerbation of seizures from high phenytoin levels, therefore, appears to be very uncommon, and fears of such increases should not discourage efforts, in most patients, to obtain maximally tolerated doses if the seizures are difficult to control.

62. Increase the phenytoin dose in 25-mg increments after a 300-mg daily dose has been achieved.

One of the most valuable antiepileptic drugs in the neurologist's armamentarium is phenytoin, and maximal effectiveness of this drug is critical to maximal seizure control of appropriate seizure types. The problem of inadequate dose is addressed in principle 61. The method of increasing the phenytoin dose is related to the size of the available capsules and tablets. The standard 100-mg capsule can be supplemented with smaller doses, either the chewable 50-mg tablet or the 30-mg capsule available in the United States.

The 50-mg tablet has certain advantages. It is half the size of the standard capsule, and makes 50-mg increments easy to organize and remember. It can be broken in half, so that the dose can be increased in 25-mg increments (e.g., 300 to 325 to 350, and so on).

A theoretical disadvantage of the 50-mg tablet is the formulation, which is different than that of the capsules. The capsules (30 or 100 mg) contain the sodium salt of phenytoin (diphenylhydantoin sodium), whereas the 50-mg chewable tablets contain the free acid of phenytoin. Although absorption of the free acid may be different than that of the sodium salt, no serious problem is encountered, provided that eventual absorption is total, which it apparently is in most patients. Another problem is the 8% increase in dose, mg for mg, of the free acid over the sodium salt. A direct conversion of four 100-mg capsules to eight 50-mg tablets would yield an equivalent of 432 mg in sodium phenytoin. Such a substitution is quite unlikely, but toxicity may result in the event of such a change. If, as in the usual case, the 50-mg tablets merely supplement the capsules in increments of 25, 50, or 75 mg, the formulation effect is negligible.

The 30-mg capsules avoid the problem of formulation differences, since they contain the sodium salt. The 30-mg incremental increase in dose is preferred by many doctors and is just as effective as using the 50-mg tablets.

63. Phenytoin and carbamazepine can be used together.

Although the mechanisms of action of phenytoin and carbamazepine are largely unknown — we do not even know whether they work by the same mechanism — they can clearly be used together with considerable clinical effectiveness. Experimentally, these two drugs are the most effective in animal models of seizures that correlate with partial and generalized tonic-clonic seizures in humans, and their combined clinical efficacy is superior to their individual efficacy (Porter et al., 1980). Neither drug has a primary sedative effect, and when used together, plasma levels of each can usually be achieved in the upper therapeutic range without toxic side effects. For patients with refractory partial seizures or generalized tonic-clonic seizures, this combination of drugs offers maximal seizure control with minimal toxicity. Occasionally, the addition of carbamazepine causes an increase in the plasma phenytoin level (Gratz et al., 1982), but such problems can be avoided by careful monitoring of the plasma drug levels. A typical regimen is outlined in principle 60.

When phenytoin and carbamazepine together fail to effect seizure control, then valproate may be added to the regimen. Although valproate appears to be ineffective in partial seizures, the evidence for the effectiveness of this drug in generalized tonic-clonic seizures is controversial. The favorable response of some patients, however, remains a possibility, and a trial of this nonsedative drug is occasionally worthwhile in patients who do not respond adequately to phenytoin and carbamazepine.

64. Watch for saturation kinetics with phenytoin.

The problem with phenytoin, a problem not shared with other antiepileptic drugs, is the relationship between dose and plasma level of the drug, which becomes more and more nonlinear as higher doses are given. The phenomenon is known as saturation or Michaelis-Menten kinetics. The body has a decreased ability to eliminate a fixed percentage of the dose administered as higher doses are given. In practical terms, it means that the half-life of the drug may be much longer at higher doses than at lower doses. Therefore, all the caveats about the clinical use of long half-life drugs become doubly important at phenytoin levels exceeding 12 to 15 μg/ml. To avoid problems with phenytoin, note the following:

1. At higher doses, the increases should be spread over long intervals to avoid the occurrence of toxicity many days later — even weeks may be necessary between dose changes (Porter et al., 1980).
2. The plasma phenytoin level may not change immediately after a dose change; the level may plateau for up to a week before further increases or decreases in the level occur spontaneously.
3. Evaluation of seizure control must be delayed until a steady-state level is achieved (principle 51).

Overall, the most common mistake in dealing with saturation kinetics is increasing the phenytoin dose every 2 or 3 days until toxicity occurs. Unfortunately, such increases are usually made long before a steady-state level is achieved. When toxicity occurs under these circumstances, it may be severe, as the plasma phenytoin level continues to increase on a constant dose. The physician may then erroneously conclude that the patient has a low tolerance for the drug. To avoid these problems, use small dose increments (principle 62), make changes slowly, and monitor plasma phenytoin levels frequently.

Patients with epilepsy are unfortunately variable in their tolerance of phenytoin. They tolerate higher doses than healthy volunteers (Jusko, 1976), but some adult epileptic patients tolerate less than 250 mg/day, whereas others easily tolerate 450 mg/day or more. Part of this difference can be explained by the heterogeneous nonlinear kinetics of various patients (Fig. 64.1). Attempts to predict doses or plasma levels of phenytoin in individual patients have met with limited success (Murphy et al., 1981), and the empirical approaches noted above are clinically still the most effective.

65. Diplopia is the most common dose-related side effect of high plasma carbamazepine levels.

Carbamazepine is the most effective nonsedative addition to the armamentarium of drugs effective against both generalized tonic-clonic seizures and partial seizures since the development of phenytoin. Double vision (diplopia) is the most common dose-related complaint of patients taking carbamazepine. It usually lasts 30 min to 2 hr, and usually begins within 1 or 2 hr after a dose. The diplopia most often can be related to a failure of the mechanisms of conjugate gaze; it usually disappears if either eye is covered, a useful test to assure the physician of the cause. Some patients complain of double vision as the plasma carbamazepine level reaches about 8 μg/ml (assuming trough levels), and rearrangement of dose can sometimes reduce toxicity without decreasing the total dose. If a patient has double vision or other dose-related side effects at a specific time of day, measurement of the plasma carbamazepine level at the time when toxic symptoms are present will help establish whether carbamazepine is the offender; such levels are

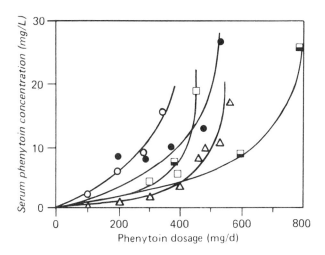

Fig 64.1. Non-linear effect of phenytoin dose on plasma phenytoin level. Five patients received increasing oral doses of phenytoin, and the steady-state level was measured at each dose. As expected from saturation kinetics, the curves are not linear; as the dose increases, the plasma phenytoin levels rise at an even more rapid rate. The patients showed marked variation in the plasma phenytoin levels achieved at the various doses. (From Porter and Pitlick, 1982; modified from Jusko, 1976, with permission).

especially useful in patients on multiple drugs. There is no evidence of a significant lag between brain and blood levels under such circumstances, and the plasma drug level will, at least proportionately, reflect the brain level.

Diplopia may be helpful in distinguishing clinically the toxic effects of carbamazepine from those of phenytoin. In the case of the latter drug, dose-related side effects usually last longer; furthermore, phenytoin toxicity usually presents with ataxia rather than double vision. Carbamazepine usually causes ataxia only at very high doses. Unfortunately, these differences between phenytoin and carbamazepine are not entirely reliable, and measurement of plasma drug levels at the time of complaint is the only sure method of identifying the offending drug when multiple drugs are involved.

Other dose-related side effects are reported to be especially prominent when carbamazepine is first administered. Drowsiness, loss of appetite, dizziness, and nausea can usually be avoided by beginning with a smaller dose and increasing it gradually to the maximally tolerated dose. Some of these toxic effects, especially dizziness, occur at lower doses in older patients.

Two dose-related side effects of carbamazepine are worthy of special mention. The drug occasionally causes hyponatremia with water intoxication. The presenting clinical complaints are usually headache and confusion, the latter if the drop in serum sodium is sudden or severe. Water retention may occur, but apparently only in the presence of decreased serum sodium. Measurement of the serum sodium level is the obvious diagnostic measure in patients suspected of having this problem. The other side effect is choreoathetosis, which is rare, and occurs at high doses (Sheridan et al., 1983). It may occur only in especially susceptible patients and, therefore, may be more idiosyncratic than dose related. Other idiosyncratic side effects of carbamazepine are described in principle 67.

66. Ataxia is a common dose-related side effect of high plasma phenytoin levels.

Phenytoin is perhaps the most widely used antiepileptic drug, effective against both generalized tonic-clonic seizures and partial seizures. Kutt et al. (1964) has analyzed the common dose-related toxicity of phenytoin. He found the following relationships between side effects and plasma phenytoin levels: (1) nystagmus begins at about 15 to 20 μg/ml, (2) ataxia begins at about 30 μg/ml, and (3) mental changes begin at about 40 μg/ml (Fig. 66.1). Nystagmus was rarely symptomatic, however, and the onset of ataxia was quite variable. Some patients had the onset of ataxia at a level of 25 μg/ml, but others were unaffected until a level of 40 μg/ml was achieved. This early study confirmed that most patients on twice a day dosage will be able to tolerate an early morning (before morning medication) level of 17 to 22 μg/ml (principle 61). Some will have nystagmus, including vertical nystagmus, and many will have interruption of smooth pursuit eye movements, but they are usually asymptomatic; there is usually no reason to change the dose.

Other dose-related side effects of phenytoin include diplopia and, rarely, acute extrapyramidal dyskinesias at very high levels. Hirsutism is a problem, especially in girls and young women. Suggestions of interference with higher cortical function and changes in behavior, while well recognized at high levels, are controversial at usual therapeutic levels.

Adverse effects of long-term use of phenytoin include gingival hyperplasia, which appears to be dose related, and peripheral neuropathy (usually decreased reflexes in the lower extremities), which may not be dose related. Cerebellar ataxia has been thought by some to be related to long-term phenytoin therapy, but the evidence is not yet convincing.

Idiosyncratic reactions to phenytoin are rare; skin rashes are the most common. Also reported are megaloblastic anemia, leukopenia, and lymphadenopathy. Hepatotoxicity and aplastic anemia are extremely uncommon. These reactions have been well reviewed (Dam, 1982; Pisciotta, 1982).

67. The most important idiosyncratic side effect of carbamazepine is hematologic.

Carbamazepine attained an early reputation in the United States as a drug with a high potential for serious hematologic toxicity. This fear delayed access of epileptic patients in the United States to this drug until its efficacy was proved unequivocally (Cereghino et al., 1974). The drug has none of the

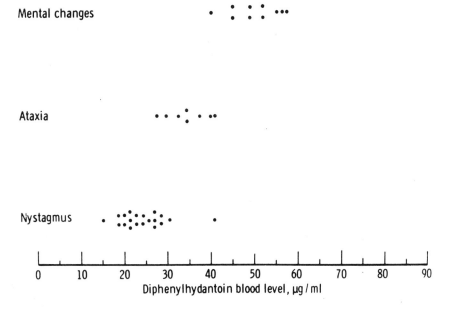

Fig. 66.1. The onset of nystagmus, ataxia, and mental changes in relation to phenytoin levels (From Kutt et al., 1964.)

sedative or adverse effects on behavior of the barbiturates and causes none of the problems associated with long-term phenytoin use.

The idiosyncratic hematologic reaction to carbamazepine is bone marrow depression, which though quite rare, can be fatal. Pisciotta (1982) reviewed 22 patients with aplastic anemia who took carbamazepine; 13 of these patients died, but the relationship to the drug was uncertain in many, and many were taking other drugs. Other hematologic reactions, such as leukopenia and agranulocytosis, were also noted, but the vast majority of the affected patients recovered from these disorders. Because many clinicians and investigators have also observed mild but persistent leukopenia during carbamazepine therapy, guidelines for monitoring hematologic function are not uniformly accepted. One possible plan, following the introduction of treatment, is to monitor the leukocyte count weekly for a month, then biweekly for an additional 6 weeks. A delicate balance must be achieved in patients who need the drug for seizure control, but who have persistent leukopenia.

Another group of idiosyncratic reactions to carbamazepine are skin rashes, which usually necessitate discontinuation of therapy. Occasionally, patients who have a history of a rash merit rechallenge with carbamazepine if seizure control is poor and the drug is deemed clinically necessary. Such a rechallenge should be done with the patient in the hospital and with the advice of a consultant allergist. Finally, hepatitis and cardiac arrhythmias have been associated anecdotally with carbamazepine therapy.

It must be emphasized that the idiosyncratic toxic reactions to carbamazepine or other drugs do *not* appear to be related to the amount of drug administered to the patient. The therapeutic plan of 'adding just a little carbamazepine' in hopes of minimizing the risks of life-threatening idiosyncratic bone marrow depression, therefore, has no rational basis. If carbamazepine is needed for seizure control, the fear of idiosyncratic reactions need not inhibit its use at high doses. The dose-related reactions to carbamazepine are reviewed in principle 65.

68. Do not give phenytoin intramuscularly.

The temptation to give phenytoin intramuscularly is most often related to a temporary inability of the patient to take oral medications, such as during surgical recovery or during vomiting episodes. Several serious problems arise with the use of this route of administration that make it an undesirable method of giving the drug. First, the drug is soluble only if the pH is maintained at 12; when the intravenous preparation is injected intramuscularly into cats, precipitation and crystallization of the drug occur, with hemorrhage into and necrosis of the muscle (Serrano and Wilder, 1974); the latter may also be related to the vehicle, propylene glycol. The crystals disappear after 24 hr. Second, seizure control is compromised by the crystallization and resultant slow absorption of the drug — the phenytoin is trapped in what is essentially a crystalline depot in the muscle. When intramuscular therapy replaces oral therapy, the result is a temporary fall in plasma phenytoin levels because of this trapping of the drug. As noted in the cat studies, however, the drug is eventually totally absorbed from the depot. If this delayed release from the depot occurs after oral therapy has been resumed, drug intoxication can result (Serrano et al., 1973).

To counter the pharmacokinetic problems noted above, Wilder and Ramsay (1976) studied the intramuscular administration of phenytoin in 12 patients. Following stabilization on an oral regimen, the patients were given phenytoin intramuscularly at a dose that was 50% higher than the oral stabilization dose. After 1 week the patients were returned, for another week, to an oral dose 50% lower than the original oral dose. Seizure control was not affected. This complex regimen requires a single daily injection of phenytoin; more frequent injections cause significant rises in the plasma phenytoin levels. Because of individual variations, monitoring of plasma phenytoin levels is recommended when attempting this complicated plan.

In summary, because of possible muscle damage and the complexities of maintaining adequate plasma drug levels, intramuscular use of phenytoin is not recommended. Phenytoin can be given, when appropriate and when aspiration is not threatened, by gastric intubation. If the gastrointestinal route is not possible, a daily intravenous injection of the drug (principle 85) is highly appropriate until the oral route of administration can be resumed.

69. Phenacemide is toxic and only rarely indicated.

Phenacemide is a ring-opened analog of phenytoin and is extremely similar to phenytoin in conformational structure (Camerman and Camerman, 1980). It is effective in experimental animals as an antiepileptic agent, but its use is severely limited in humans by its idiosyncratic toxicity, which may occur in as many as 30% of patients (Troupin, 1976). The drug is only indicated after other antiepileptic drugs have failed, and even then the significant risks often outweigh the potential benefits.

The personality changes associated with phenacemide use are difficult to manage. Depression may be associated with suicide attempts, and aggressive behavior may also occur. Patients with a history of personality disorders should be considered for treatment with phenacemide only if hospitalized during the initial treatment.

Organ toxicity is also common. Fatal hepatotoxicity has been reported, as has fatal aplastic anemia. Nephritis has also been reported.

One of the interesting aspects of phenacemide is the rather high doses that are considered tolerable and effective. Two or three grams are considered an average daily dose, and some adult patients tolerate as much as 5 g/day.

Because of its toxicity, no studies have established the role of phenacemide in the antiepileptic drug armamentarium. Unknown, therefore, is information on the uniqueness of patients who might respond to the drug. It should be used sparingly and with extreme caution. Plasma phenacemide levels are not generally available for clinical use.

70. Mephenytoin has a limited therapeutic role.

Mephenytoin is metabolized to an active metabolite, 5-ethyl-5-phenylhydantoin (Nirvanol), which was marketed in the 1920's and early 1930's for the treatment of chorea (primarily Sydenham's chorea). Studies by Jones and Jacobs (1932) and others, however, demonstrated that Nirvanol had little efficacy in chorea and, furthermore, that it caused fever, rash, eosinophilia, thrombocytopenia and bleeding. For these reasons, Nirvanol was withdrawn from the market.

The antiepileptic drug mephenytoin was not marketed in the United States until the mid-1940's. Various uncontrolled studies suggest that it has some efficacy in generalized tonic-clonic seizures and partial seizures. Mephenytoin is still available in the United States and some other countries.

Relatively recent studies in humans show that Nirvanol may be responsible for most of the antiepileptic activity of mephenytoin (Kupferberg et al., 1978). Mephenytoin has a mean half-life of 14 to 15 hr, whereas Nirvanol has a mean half-life of 3 or 4 days. Furthermore, the average steady-state plasma mephenytoin level is only 1.5 μg/ml, whereas the average plasma Nirvanol level is 18 μg/ml in patients taking a 400-mg daily dose of mephenytoin (Kupferberg, 1982). In mice, moreover, Nirvanol is actually more potent against maximal electroshock seizures than is mephenytoin (Kupferberg and Yonekawa, 1975). When the doctor prescribes mephenytoin, therefore, the major pharmacologically active drug appears to be Nirvanol, not the parent compound.

If the metabolite Nirvanol is the pharmacologically active agent derived from mephenytoin, and if Nirvanol was removed from the market almost half a century ago because of its toxicity, the documentation of mephenytoin toxicity is clearly of great importance. The most serious side effect of mephenytoin is bone marrow depression. In a review by Robins (1962), 25 cases of aplastic anemia were associated with the use of mephenytoin as the sole drug, resulting in 16 deaths. Additional cases also suggested mephenytoin-induced aplastic anemia, but the patients were receiving other medications. The frequency of skin rashes is also apparently higher than for phenytoin, although such comparisons are difficult to make because of the anecdotal nature of the reports.

Many of the dose-related side effects of mephenytoin, such as nystagmus, diplopia, and ataxia, appear to be similar to those of phenytoin, but mephenytoin apparently does not cause hirsutism, gingival hyperplasia, or peripheral neuropathy (Troupin et al., 1976), all of which have been associated with phenytoin.

In summary, the role of mephenytoin appears to be limited primarily by its toxicity. Convincing evidence of its superior efficacy, as compared with phenytoin, is not available. Because plasma levels of mephenytoin or Nirvanol cannot be obtained except in research centers, use of mephenytoin is rarely warranted.

CHAPTER ELEVEN

Therapy: Generalized Seizures

71. Use carbamazepine and/or phenytoin for generalized tonic-clonic seizures.

The treatment of generalized tonic-clonic seizures is similar to that of partial seizures (see Chapter 10). Carbamazepine and/or phenytoin are the current drugs of choice. These drugs are especially effective when used together (principle 63). The reason for the effectiveness of these drugs is not known, but it may well be related to the likelihood that most generalized tonic-clonic attacks are secondary to partial seizures (principle 23).

There are some patients whose generalized tonic-clonic seizures do not respond to a regimen of these two drugs. Experimentally, neither carbamazepine nor phenytoin are effective against threshold seizure tests in rodents, suggesting that patients who are unresponsive to these drugs may have primary generalized seizures. In support of this concept, control of generalized tonic-clonic seizures occurring secondary to partial seizures is relatively easy, whereas control of apparently primary generalized tonic-clonic seizures is often difficult. For patients with primary generalized tonic-clonic seizures, valproate may be of some value. One study (Turnbull et al., 1982) suggests that valproate is equally as effective as phenytoin in the treatment of generalized tonic-clonic seizures, but conclusive data are not yet available.

The use of barbiturates for the control of generalized tonic-clonic seizures is rarely necessary, considering the effectiveness and nonsedative characteristics of phenytoin, carbamazepine, and valproate. Benzodiazepines are usually ineffective in the long-term treatment of generalized tonic-clonic attacks, and are rarely indicated.

Patients who have had only a single generalized tonic-clonic seizure and whose evaluation (medical history, neurologic examination, and usually an EEG and a CT scan) otherwise reveals no abnormalities are not usually considered to have epilepsy and require no therapy (Marsden, 1976). Although some of these patients will later have another seizure, no investigations can identify them before the second seizure occurs.

72. The response to antiabsence medication can be quantified.

Most seizure types are not associated with characteristic EEG changes that allow quantification of seizure frequency by use of the EEG alone. The subtle slowing of a temporal lobe focus in the EEG of a patient with complex partial seizures, for example, may be helpful in establishing the seizure diagnosis in the individual patient, but the abnormality does not correlate sufficiently with the clinical occurrence of complex partial seizures to allow EEG quantification of seizure frequency.

Absence seizures, on the other hand, are characteristically associated with generalized, high voltage, spike-and-wave discharges in the EEG; these abnormal waveforms usually occur at 2.5 to 3.5 Hz. A large number of behavioral measures, reviewed by Penry (1973), have shown that performance is decreased during the spike-and-wave discharge. In early studies it was difficult to control the timing of the performance tests, as it was not possible to insert a performance task at a precise moment in the spike-and-wave paroxysm in order to evaluate responsiveness. This difficulty was overcome by causing the abnormal EEG discharge to trigger a reaction-time stimulus (Porter et al., 1973), using a simple amplitude detector on one channel of the EEG machine. A total of 235 spike-and-wave discharges were studied in 14 patients, and 56% of the stimuli delivered at the onset of the spike-and-wave burst resulted in abnormal responses (Porter et al., 1973). These studies were extended by Browne et al. (1974), who introduced a 0.5 sec delay after the onset of the spike-and-wave discharge before the stimulus was delivered (Fig. 72.1). The reaction times before, during, and after spike-and-wave paroxysms in 26 patients are shown in Fig. 72.2.

Several important conclusions may be drawn from these studies. First, generalized spike-and-wave paroxysms in the EEG are highly correlated with a decrement in consciousness. The generalized spike-and-wave abnormality, therefore, unlike most electrographic abnormalities, correlates directly with the seizure itself, and obviously the number of generalized spike-and-wave paroxysms will give an excellent estimate of the seizure frequency. A decrement in consciousness occurs even if the paroxysm is brief (i.e., lasts less than 2 to 3 sec). Second, although efforts have been made to automate the counting of such events (Ehrenberg and Penry, 1976), most studies have utilized hand counting of the discharges. For the doctor treating a patient with absence seizures, a long-term EEG recording before and after each medication change will help to assess the effectiveness of therapy. For the clinical investigator, the availability of an objective and recordable method for determining seizure frequency is extremely useful (principle 73).

The final important observation from these studies of responsiveness relates to the cerebral distribution of the abnormal spike-and-wave discharges. Completely generalized discharges were highly correlated with altered consciousness. Incompletely generalized discharges caused lesser impairment of responsiveness, although the likelihood of some impairment was still high. (Browne et al., 1974).

In conclusion, antiabsence therapy should be aimed at elimination of not only clinical seizures but also as many generalized spike-and-wave discharges as possible. Many brief absence attacks may go unnoticed clinically, and the EEG is the best way to identify such seizures. This is the only seizure type in which 'treating the EEG' has a highly rational basis.

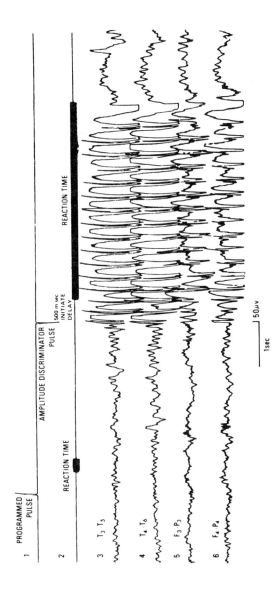

Fig. 72.1. Recording from a six-channel polygraph showing reaction time with a 0.5-sec delay from the time of onset of generalized spike-and-wave discharge to the time of auditory stimulus. The amplitude discriminator (threshold detector) monitored channel four and triggered the stimulus when the EEG amplitude exceeded 100 μV. In this case, the patient responded with a normal reaction time 3 sec before the paroxysm, but was unable to respond after the paroxysm began; unresponsiveness persisted until the paroxysm ended. (From Browne et al., 1974.)

73. Ethosuximide is the drug of choice for absence seizures.

Recognition of absence seizures is important in part because of the effective treatments available. Ethosuximide has been the drug of choice for the treatment of absence attacks since its introduction in 1960. The drug is relatively nontoxic and nonsedative.

The effectiveness of ethosuximide has been documented in a single-blind study using multiple criteria for determination of efficacy (Browne et al., 1975). In 37 patients receiving the drug, 49% achieved at least 90% control of their attacks and 95% achieved at least 50% control. Sherwin et al. (1973) undertook a similar study which showed not only that about 75% of absence seizure patients could gain seizure control, but also that monitoring of plasma drug levels was very useful, improving both the effective dose and the patients' compliance (Fig. 73.1).

Although previous studies had suggested that ethosuximide might worsen behavior in children who took the drug, 17 of 37 patients actually improved in a blind study with matched controls; only one patient was worse (Browne et al., 1975).

The effect of ethosuximide occurs rapidly. In 18 patients with long-term telemetered EEG recordings, the most impressive decline in spike-and-wave bursts was seen in the first 48 hr of therapy (Penry et al., 1972).

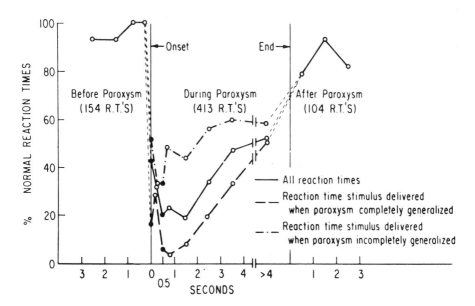

Fig. 72.2. Graph of 671 reaction times (R.T.'s) from 26 patients showing percentages of normal reaction times before, during, and after spike-and-wave paroxysms. Patients were least responsive when the paroxysms were completely generalized. There is no evidence of a decrement in consciousness before the onset of the paroxysms, and patients are normally responsive only 2 sec after the end of the attack. (From Browne et al., 1974.)

The effective plasma ethosuximide level is rarely less than 60 μg/ml and extends to at least 100 μg/ml. Some feel that, for resistant patients, further improvements may be observed at even higher levels, occasionally as high as 150 μg/ml (Sherwin, 1982). The drug has a long half-life, but spacing of the doses during the day is necessary more for the avoidance of gastrointestinal side effects than for achievement of a smooth steady-state level (principle 51). As with other antiepileptic drugs, ethosuximide should be utilized vigorously and fully before being abandoned as ineffective. Occasionally, a small dose of ethosuximide is added to an already complex antiepileptic drug regimen. Such use almost always fails, and may give a false impression that the drug is not efficacious.

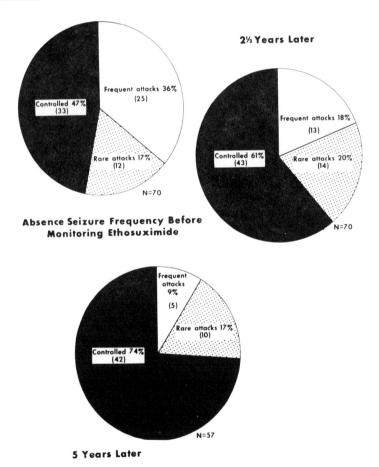

Fig. 73.1. The control of absence attacks before monitoring plasma drug levels and 2½ and 5 years after commencing monitoring. The improvements were highly significant and greatly in excess of what might have been expected from the natural course of remission of absence attacks. Nineteen patients of the original 70 had significant increases in plasma ethosuximide levels after 2½ years; 13 of these had improved seizure control, including 10 who became seizure free. (From Sherwin, 1982.)

The chief dose-related side effects of ethosuximide are nausea, vomiting, and anorexia. Initial drowsiness rarely persists. These side effects necessitate a regimen which includes a gradual build-up of the drug. Although 1,500 to 2,000 mg daily may be the dose necessary eventually to achieve seizure control, treatment may need to begin slowly, with 250 to 500 mg/day initially. Gastrointestinal side effects can often be alleviated by temporary dose reduction; dose increases are often possible later.

Bone marrow depression is an exceedingly rare idiosyncratic side effect of ethosuximide, but it can be fatal. Monthly blood counts are recommended (Dreifuss, 1982), but most of the cases have occurred within 6 months of the initiation of therapy. Other side effects include skin rashes and lupus-like reactions. Psychosis has also been reported, but as with other idiosyncratic reactions to ethosuximide, it is unusual, and may occur only in predisposed patients.

Ethosuximide is also the drug of choice for the long-term treatment of absence status and for the related forms of petit mal status epilepticus, for which no descriptive term is really adequate (Porter and Penry, 1983). Valproate is also highly effective in many such patients. The acute attacks can usually be terminated with intravenously administered diazepam, if necessary.

74. Valproate is highly effective for absence seizures.

Absence seizures respond well not only to ethosuximide but also to valproate, a relatively new drug. This compound was accidentally discovered as it was being used as a vehicle to test potential antiepileptic drugs. The vehicle was shown to have antiepileptic potency by itself, and a new drug was discovered serendipitously for the treatment of epilepsy. Valproate has been marketed in the United States since 1978. It is available as a 250-mg capsule of valproic acid in corn oil and as a syrup of sodium valproate; 5 ml (one teaspoon) of the latter is equivalent to one 250-mg capsule of the free acid, making conversion simple. At least three forms of valproate are now marketed (Fig. 74.1). In countries where sodium valproate is marketed in tablet form, it is enclosed in foil, as it is very hygroscopic; the tablets usually contain 250 mg of sodium valproate. Magnesium valproate is available in Latin America; it comes in tablets that are not very hygroscopic and do not require foil wrappers. Calcium valproate may soon be available, and a valproate formulation has been designed for enteric release to alleviate some of the gastrointestinal side effects.

Valproate is highly effective against absence seizures (Simon and Penry, 1975) and decreases the generalized spike-and-wave paroxysms that accompany such attacks (Penry et al., 1976). With the use of 12-hr telemetered EEGs to measure the frequency of generalized spike-and-wave discharges, valproate was compared with ethosuximide in a double-blind, response-conditional crossover study of absence seizures in 45 patients (Sato et al., 1982). Valproate was equally as effective as ethosuximide. Patients who meet the diagnostic criteria for absence seizures and who do not respond to ethosuximide should be considered for treatment with valproate. The drug should be started in relatively low doses, with gradual build-up to a therapeutic level. Valproate shares with ethosuximide a tendency to irritate the gastrointestinal tract. This tendency can usually be overcome with slowly increasing doses and considerable patience.

Valproate is also effective against certain myclonias (principle 82) and may be effective against generalized tonic-clonic seizures (principle 71).

The dose of valproate necessary for seizure control is often more than 30 mg/kg. In some patients, doses of 60 mg/kg are required to reach reasonable plasma valprote levels and maximal efficacy. The therapeutic level (before the morning dose — see principle 54) ranges from 60 to 100 μg/ml, but every effort should be made to exceed 80 μg/ml before abandoning the drug in resistant cases. Many patients, furthermore, tolerate levels considerably higher than 100 μg/ml. As higher doses are approached, it should be recognized that the drug has a short half-life and that a four-times-a-day dosing regimen will allow maximum daily dosage with minimal side effects (principle 49). Some of the gastrointestinal side effects, which appear to be more severe with the free acid than the salt, may be alleviated by the newer enteric-coated formulation.

Some side effects are unique to valproate. Weight gain is a problem in a small percentage of patients, presumably from increased appetite. Hair loss is temporary and reversible on dose reduction or discontinuation, but may be dramatic in a few affected patients. A fine tremor occurs at higher doses.

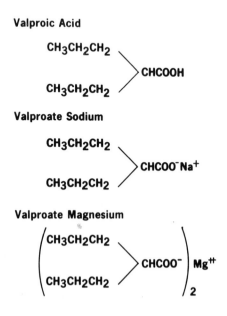

Fig. 74.1.   Three of the most common forms of valproate (see text).

Reversible amenorrhea has been noted. Platelet decreases are reported, but bleeding is not a sufficiently well-documented side effect to cause concern.

Another dose-related side effect of valproate is its interaction with other drugs. No other antiepileptic drug has presented the potential difficulties with drug-drug interaction that arise with valproate. The two most notable interactions are with phenobarbital and phenytoin. The more important is the interaction with phenobarbital, in which the level of the barbiturate may suddenly rise, resulting in stupor, coma, or even psychosis. Kapetanovic et al. (1981) studied this interaction in three patients who were taking only phenobarbital. A single pulse-dose of stable isotope-labeled phenobarbital was given at steady-state plasma phenobarbital levels (Kapetanovic et al., 1980). The half-lives of phenobarbital in these patients ranged from 61 to 135 hr. Following administration of valproate in doses ranging from 1,500 to 2,000 mg/day, the plasma phenobarbital levels rose, but the excretion of the metabolite, hydroxyphenobarbital, decreased. When another pulse of isotopically labeled phenobarbital was given, the half-lives of phenobarbital had increased to a range of 94 to 163 hr. The main effect of valproate on phenobarbital, therefore, appears to be inhibition of phenobarbital metabolism. Patients who are taking phenobarbital, especially those with plasma phenobarbital levels of more than 25 μg/ml, should have valproate added to their regimen only with considerable caution and with attention to changes in the phenobarbital level.

A less important and different interaction is a valproate-induced decrease in phenytoin levels. Whether the decrement in phenytoin levels is clinically significant is debatable, but a concomitant rise in free phenytoin levels may counteract any decrease in total levels. Studies of binding of the two drugs suggest mutual displacement from plasma proteins (Cramer and Mattson, 1979).* Only rarely does the interaction between valproate and phenytoin require regimen changes.

One regrettable, life-threatening side effect of valproate is acute hepatotoxicity (Suchy et al., 1979). The evidence is strong that this side effect is idiosyncratic and not dose-related. In a series of 25 patients reported by the manufacturer, the fatal hepatotoxicity did not appear to have any specific relation to age or dose (Table 74.1). Although the serum glutamic oxaloacetic transaminase (SGOT) may return to normal in some patients if the drug is stopped, the clinical course appears to be inexorable in others. Furthermore, the SGOT may not rise dramatically and is a limited predictor of eventual outcome; it is, nevertheless, the best biochemical monitoring technique available and should be followed closely for the first 6 months of therapy. The hepatotoxicity may present with malaise, sleepiness, vomiting and jaundice.

---

*Only two antiepileptic drugs, phenytoin and valproate, are bound to plasma proteins to a degree to be of even theoretical clinical importance. While considerable data are available on the degree of binding of these two drugs in various conditions, the clinical utility of determining free levels of these drugs remains uncertain except in specific conditions, such as uremia or hypoalbuminemia (Porter and Layzer, 1975).

Table 74.1.   Twenty-five patients with fatal hepatotoxicity associated with valproate

Age: 5 months to 28 years
Dose: 10 to 90 mg/kg/day
Time lapse from initiation of therapy: 3 to 180 days
First abnormal SGOT: 34 to 564 mU/ml
Highest SGOT before death: 128 to 12,000 mU/ml

Compiled from data supplied by Abbott Laboratories, 1981.

75.   Ethosuximide and valproate can be used together.

Both ethosuximide and valproate offer effective and nonsedative therapy for absence seizures. It is likely that these two different drugs suppress seizures by different mechanisms. More important clinically, however, the drugs are effective when used together to treat absence seizures. This effectiveness may have an important impact on patients who are resistant to one drug or the other. Whenever possible, patients with intractable absence seizures should be given both drugs at the same time. Such a trial is especially important in this particular seizure type, since therapy of absence attacks is, overall, often effective. Plasma levels of both drugs may exceed to 60 to 80 μg/ml, although some patients may not require maximal doses of both drugs to achieve complete control.

Clonazepam and nitrazepam are also effective against absence seizures. Clonazepam is an extremely potent antiepileptic drug. Its plasma level is measured in nanograms instead of micrograms. Unfortunately, these benzodiazepines are rarely indicated because of dose-related side effects (principle 86) and must be reserved for patients who cannot tolerate the two nonsedative drugs. Patients whose seizures are refractory to ethosuximide and/or valproate will only rarely derive overall improvement from the benzodiazepines. Clonazepam has little proven effectiveness other than for absence seizures.

The effectiveness of barbiturates in absence seizure therapy is, at best, exceedingly limited. The most undesirable side effect of these drugs, sedation, can actually worsen absence seizure frequency (Penry and So, 1981). The use of barbiturates in the treatment of epilepsy is discussed in Chapter 13.

76.   Phensuximide is generally ineffective.

There are three marketed succinimides that are potentially useful for absence seizures. These are phensuximide, methsuximide, and ethosuximide. The first of these, phensuximide, was marketed in the United States in 1953 and was the first alternative to the more toxic diones (principle 78). The drug was initially greeted with enthusiasm, but within a few years was noted to be less potent than trimethadione and has never been completely accepted as an effective agent.

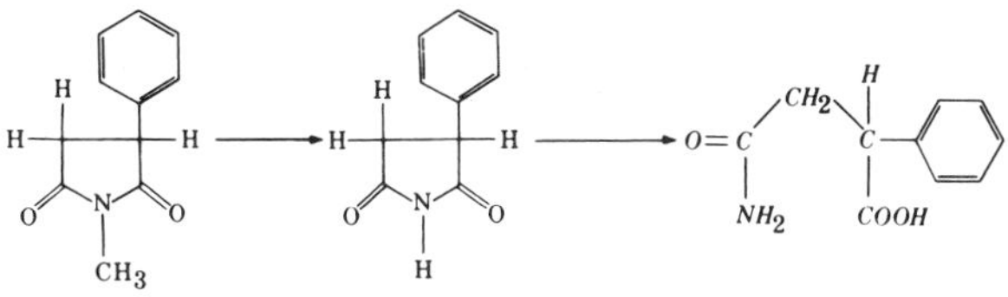

Phensuximide   Desmethylphensuximide   Phenylsuccinamic acid

Fig. 76.1.   Phensuximide is rapidly metabolized to an inactive compound. It is first demethylated to desmethylphensuximide and then quickly converted to phenylsuccinamic acid by ring opening. (From Porter and Kupferberg, 1982.)

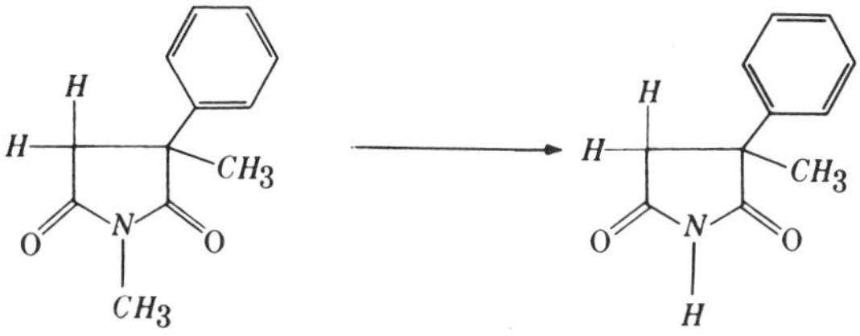

Methsuximide   Desmethylmethsuximide

Fig. 76.2.   Methsuximide is rapidly converted to desmethylmethsuximide, but further metabolism is slow. Accumulation of the desmethylmethsuximide accounts for the antiepileptic efficacy of the drug. (From Porter and Kupferberg, 1982.)

In the past few years, a fundamental pharmacologic reason for the ineffectiveness of phensuximide has been documented (Porter et al., 1979). Neither the drug nor its demethylated metabolite, desmethylphensuximide, (Fig. 76.1) accumulate to any significant extent in the body. The rapid removal of the metabolite is most probably due to the action of a liver enzyme, dihydropyrimidinase, which opens the succinimide ring and quickly inactivates desmethylphensuximide. This enzyme cannot open the ring in desmethylmethsuximide because of the protection provided by the additional methyl group (Fig. 76.2). Since the ring-opened compound is apparently inactive, no effective antiepileptic drug accumulates. The use of phensuximide, therefore, is not recommended. Methsuximide, however, which is metabolized differently, is occasionally an effective alternative to ethosuximide.

77. Methsuximide is more toxic than ethosuximide, but may have a broader spectrum of activity.

Methsuximide has a short half-life, and its desmethyl metabolite is primarily responsible for the drug's efficacy (principle 76). Steady-state levels of the metabolite, although rarely measured, are usually in the range of 20 to

40 μg/ml, with a half-life of 28 to 58 hr (Porter et al., 1979). Experimentally, methsuximide has a broader range of effectiveness than that of ethosuximide. The former is active against pentylenetetrazol-induced seizures as well as maximal electroshock (MES) convulsions in mice. Ethosuximide, on the other hand, is a 'pure' antiabsence drug, effective experimentally only against pentylenetetrazol-induced seizures, and clinically only against absence seizures.

To evaluate the possible role of methsuximide in partial seizures (which would correlate with the MES activity of the drug), Wilder and Buchanan (1981) studied 21 outpatients with well-documented complex partial seizures, adding methsuximide to current therapy. Improvement in seizure control was impressive in 71% of the patients. Only dose-related side effects were encountered. Unfortunately, the study was not carried out blind, and the placebo effect, which may be significant in drug trials, was uncontrolled. Others have not found the drug to be as effective, and more controlled data are needed before a definitive conclusion can be reached regarding the clinical spectrum of activity of methsuximide.

Methsuximide is unquestionably effective against absence seizures. The drug's dose-related side effects, however, are more prominent than those of ethosuximide. Drowsiness, nausea, anorexia, headaches, hiccoughs, and dizziness are reported; severe idiosyncratic reactions, however, do not appear to be common (Porter and Kupferberg, 1982). Wilder and Buchanan (1981) recommended maintaining plasma levels of the desmethyl metabolite in the range of 20 to 24 μg/ml to obtain efficacy without prominent side effects.

78. Trimethadione is rarely indicated.

The first marketed antiepileptic drug effective against absence attacks was trimethadione, introduced clinically by Lennox in 1945. The drug was tested in 50 patients with 'petit mal and myoclonic and akinetic epilepsy'; 80% responded to some degree. The drug has demonstrated effectiveness and was, with its analog paramethadione, the only medication available for absence seizures until the appearance of the succinimides almost a decade later. Trimethadione is more effective than the weakest succinimide, phensuximide (principle 76), and it was not until the availability of ethosuximide that the diones were no longer necessary as primary therapy. With the advent of valproate, the use of the diones is now even less common.

The reason for limited use of the diones is not lack of efficacy (although effectiveness has not been documented by modern techniques) but rather the associated side effects. These include hemaralopia (impairment of visual acuity at high light levels) and other dose-related side effects such as sedation, fatigue, dizziness, and ataxia (Booker, 1982b). Idiosyncratic reactions include, most commonly, skin rashes, as well as bone marrow depression, and nephrotic syndrome. The drug is thought to have more teratogenic potential than most antiepileptic drugs and should not be used during pregnancy.

As with other antiepileptic drugs such as mephenytoin and methsuximide, trimethadione is rapidly converted to a long-acting metabolite, which exerts the principal antiepileptic effect. Specifically, trimethadione is demethylated to dimethadione, and steady-state studies in humans have demonstrated a 20-fold ratio of dimethadione to trimethadione (Booker, 1982a). Plasma levels of dimethadione are rarely monitored, but levels ranging from 470 to 1200 μg/ml have been correlated with seizure reduction (Booker, 1982a).

79. Absence seizures associated with generalized tonic-clonic seizures require more than ethosuximide.

One-third of patients with absence seizures have an occasional generalized tonic-clonic seizure (principle 27). These patients require specific therapy for the generalized tonic-clonic seizures, which fortunately are almost always less frequent in patients with absence seizures than in patients with partial seizures. Patients who have absence seizures but have never had a generalized tonic-clonic attack should not be given prophylactic treatment against the latter.

Ethosuximide has no beneficial effect on generalized tonic-clonic seizures, and anecdotal reports that such seizures worsen with this drug are unconfirmed. Before valproate became available, most patients with both absence seizures and generalized tonic-clonic seizures required either phenytoin or carbamazepine in addition to ethosuximide. Such a regimen is still effective, but the appropriate therapeutic plan is less obvious with the availability of valproate. Valproate has a broader spectrum of activity than ethosuximide, and may have some effectiveness against generalized tonic-clonic attacks. Some neurologists, therefore, are content to treat a patient who has both absence seizures and generalized tonic-clonic seizures with valproate alone. If the generalized tonic-clonic attacks are severe, frequent, or occur in the presence of adequate plasma valproate levels, the addition of carbamazepine or phenytoin (the former is preferred in most cases) may be prudent.

It remains an unproven, though attractive, hypothesis that controlling the absence attacks completely will cause the generalized tonic-clonic seizures to cease as well, assuming that the latter occur only secondarily to the absence attacks (principle 23). The hypothesis is difficult to test because the frequency of generalized tonic-clonic seizures in patients with absence seizures is usually low and data are difficult to obtain.

80. Acetazolamide is rarely effective.

Acetazolamide is briefly effective, especially in absence seizures, but tolerance develops, usually within a month or so, and the drug loses its effectiveness. To what extent the antiepileptic activity and/or the tolerance are related to the carbonic anhydrase activity remains uncertain. Woodbury and Kemp (1982) have concluded that the drug acts as an antiepileptic agent by inhibiting carbonic anhydrase in the glial cells of the brain; this inhibition causes an accumulation of carbon dioxide, which in turn blocks the spread of seizure activity.

There is some anecdotal evidence that acetazolamide may be useful, in a few patients, in decreasing catamenial seizures (Newmark and Penry, 1980). Tolerance does not develop if the drug is given intermittently, that is, only during the week or so before the menses, ceasing just as the menses end. Acetazolamide has a half-life of several days, so the drug will take at least 10 days to reach steady state, and the effect will persist for several days after discontinuation. The usual adult dose is 500 mg/day. No correlation between plasma acetazolamide levels and seizure control has been accomplished. Side effects are rare; of these, skin rashes are most common.

Another drug, medroxyprogesterone, has been reported to be useful in catamenial seizures (Mattson et al., 1982). Further data are needed, however, before definitive conclusions are possible regarding its efficacy.

81. Atonic seizures are highly resistant to therapy.

Seizures characterized by sudden loss of postural tone, atonic seizures (principal 28), are very difficult to treat. There is no good medical therapy for them, and surgical treatment is ineffective. The most important contribution of the neurologist is to determine the nature of other, associated seizure types, of which the atonic attacks may, in fact, be only one component. The following case report exemplifies the problem:

> A 6-year-old girl was well until the age of 5 years, when she had a generalized tonic-clonic seizure at the time of an earache and a temperature of 103°F. Lumbar puncture revealed normal CSF. Following a second generalized tonic-clonic seizure 3 weeks later, she was started on phenobarbital, which was later changed to mephobarbital because of severe hyperactivity. The generalized tonic-clonic seizures did not recur, but within a month she began having attacks of bilateral clonic twitching of the face and sudden falling; alteration of consciousness was also apparent. These attacks, which would last from 5 to 15 sec, occurred 10 to 15 times a day. One atonic attack caused a head injury with brief loss of consciousness. Phenytoin and clonazepam were added without improvement. A neurologist specializing in epilepsy saw the patient. He added valproate to the regimen and gradually discontinued all other medications. The withdrawal period was associated with some increased seizures, but the plan, executed over 6 months, was entirely successful. The child became seizure free on valproate alone.

Unfortunately, the most severe atonic attacks are much less responsive than those in the fortunate patient described above. Simon and Penry (1975) reviewed the effectiveness of the most promising drug, valproate, by combining reports on patients who were described as having either atonic or akinetic seizures. Of the 39 patients so classified (and little doubt exists that this series was heterogeneous), half had virtually no improvement from valproate and a quarter had equivocal improvement; the remaining quarter reportedly had an improvement in seizure frequency of 75% or better. The difficulty of combining results from various clinical trials to determine specific therapy for an individual patient has been emphasized (Porter & Penry, 1977; Porter, 1982; Porter, 1983a), and the difficulty is magnified in this seizure type because of classification difficulties.

Jeavons (1977) combined atonic seizures ('drop attacks'), atonic seizures with myoclonic jerks, and 'sagging' attacks and called the disorder 'myoclonic astatic epilepsy.' Of 32 such patients treated with valproate, eight became seizure free and 16 had a marked improvement in seizure frequency (Jeavons et al., 1977).

Other drugs are less effective than valproate, and some, such as clonazepam, may even worsen the atonic components of the attacks (Masland, 1975). Some patients may be better without specific therapy than with drugs that add toxicity but little efficacy (principle 86).

In summary, the patient with atonic attacks can only hope that (1) the attacks are part of another seizure type which is more responsive to therapy, (2) valproate will be effective, (3) the attacks will spontaneously remit, or (4) more effective new drugs will become available.

82. Some myoclonic seizures respond dramatically to valproate.

The myoclonias are exceedingly heterogeneous and difficult to classify (principle 29). Any reports of effectiveness of therapy in myoclonic epilepsy, therefore, must be accompanied by a description of the disorder. Simon and Penry (1975) reviewed 35 patients from several reported studies and concluded that 21 of these patients with 'myoclonic epilepsy' had an excellent response to valproate. What is not known is how many of these patients had, for example, absence seizures with myoclonic components; probably the valproate suppressed the absence attacks and the myoclonia disappeared.

Valproate does appear to have a unique role in treating certain myoclonic seizures that are distinct entities and in which other therapies are, at best, poorly effective. One such syndrome of myoclonic seizures is 'benign adolescent myoclonus' (principle 30). Valproate was reported to give excellent control of both the myoclonic jerks and the associated generalized tonic-clonic seizures in most of 11 patients with this syndrome (Ascanope and Penry, 1983).

Anecdotal evidence suggests that other myoclonic syndromes also respond uniquely to valproate. Unverricht-Lundborg syndrome, for example, appears to be unaffected in its overall prognosis, but the myoclonic symptoms can often be dramatically relieved by the drug. Other, more unusual myoclonias may also respond.

In severely affected patients, occasional use of other drugs is necessary to control the myoclonic jerks. The addition of benzodiazepines such as clonazepam, especially in combination with valproate, are especially effective in such cases, although the development of tolerance to the benzodiazepines limits their effectiveness, and the side effects are considerable. In postanoxic myoclonus, the use of L-5-hydroxy-tryptophane has been recommended (Van Woert and Rosenbaum, 1979).

In summary, many patients whose myoclonic seizures were considered refractory before the availability of valproate have responded to therapy with this drug. Which specific myoclonic attacks are responsive or unresponsive is not yet established; most such patients, therefore, deserve a trial of the drug.

83. Infantile spasms may respond to ACTH or steroids.

The treatment of infantile spasms can be quite rewarding from the standpoint of seizure control. Unfortunately, the impressive discovery that ACTH could ameliorate the epileptic attacks was followed by the disappointing observation that the drug has little or no effect on the associated mental retardation, which occurs in at least 90% of patients.

The first effective treatment for infantile spasms (principle 31) was ACTH, and many consider that it remains the drug of choice. Many different regimens have been recommended, but there is little evidence that a high dose, such as 120 to 160 units/day is more effective than a more modest dose of 20 to 40 units/day (Riikonen, 1982). Typically, patients are given daily injections for 4 to 6 weeks, with a repeat course if relapse occurs. The most common side effects, which may require either decreased dosage or discontinuation of the drug, are hypertension, Cushingoid signs, infections, and fluid retention. Although some have advocated ACTH therapy on an emergency basis in the hope of preventing uncontrolled seizures or mental retardation, evidence that this approach is effective is lacking. An amelioration of seizures is noted in approximately 60% of patients, although some will require another course of the drug to maintain the good response (Riikonen, 1982). The seizure control may be better in patients without demonstrable brain abnormalities (Lerman and Kivity, 1982).

The role of corticosteroids in infantile spasms is controversial. Many investigators feel that ACTH must be given as the primary therapy and that orally administered steroids are less effective. Others feel that the steroids are equally effective and have fewer side effects; the mode of therapy is clearly preferable to the injections of ACTH. The question can only be adequately answered by a double-blind clinical trial, using the quantification techniques developed by Frost et al. (1978). Such studies are underway. At the moment, little evidence exists for preferring one mode of therapy to the other. Some patients may respond to the alternate therapy, however, and both treatments probably should be tried in difficult cases. A course of corticosteroids is typically undertaken with either prednisone (2 mg/kg/day) or dexamethasone (0.3 mg/kg/day).

Even less is known about the role of other forms of treatment in infantile spasms. Most often used are the benzodiazepines, especially nitrazepam (not available in the Unite States) or clonazepam. Trials are underway to attempt to establish the usefulness of nitrazepam in this disorder. In most cases, these drugs are added after ACTH and corticosteroids have failed. Dose-related side effects are frequent and troublesome (principle 86). Doses of nitrazepam usually range from 0.6 to 1.0 mg/kg/day; doses of clonazepam are usually 0.1 to 0.3 mg/kg/day. Some clinicians who have access to both nitrazepam and clonazepam prefer the former.

In summary, it is suggested that a course of ACTH or a corticosteroid be given to children with infantile spasms. The course may be repeated, but toxic side effects must be carefully balanced against the benefits derived. Families should receive emotional support, but a realistic approach to the likelihood of subnormal mental development is necessary. The role of benzodiazepines is limited, and the sedative side effects may easily offset any gains in seizure control.

CHAPTER TWELVE

Therapy: Status Epilepticus

84. The two extremes of convulsive status epilepticus require different therapeutic approaches.

The treatment of generalized tonic-clonic (grand mal) status epilepticus depends on the severity of the presentation. Occasionally, the patient will present with persistent, or nearly persistent, tonic-clonic activity which is bilateral and severe. Control of such seizure activity demands minute-to-minute emergency efforts. More commonly, the patient presents with a short *history* of having had a series of tonic-clonic seizures; perhaps one attack has been observed by the emergency room physician. The seizures are separated by prolonged stuporous periods. These periods may be the predominant clinical presentation when the seizures are separated by intervals of 20 to 30 min or more.

In either case, certain life-support measures are necessary. These include maintenance of satisfactory cardiorespiratory function and monitoring of respiration, blood pressure, and the electrocardiogram. An intravenous catheter should be inserted, and blood samples should be obtained for chemistry tests, including blood urea nitrogen, electrolytes, calcium, magnesium, and glucose, as well as complete blood cell counts and determinations of plasma antiepileptic drug levels. Arterial blood gases should also be monitored (Delgado-Escueta et al., 1982). Thiamine followed by glucose should be given intravenously if alcoholism or hypoglycemia is suspected. Appropriate efforts should be made to determine the etiology of the status epilepticus.

In patients who are having continuous generalized tonic-clonic seizures, the therapy of choice is immediate intravenous administration of diazepam, beginning with 5 to 10 mg, given at a maximum rate of 10 mg/min, with the objective of stopping the attacks. Up to 20 mg can be given to an adult. As soon as the tonic-clonic activity has momentarily ceased, begin loading with an intravenous injection of phenytoin (principle 85). The anticonvulsant effect of intravenously administered diazepam is relatively short — usually only 20 to 30 min — but highly effective in most cases. The drug does have a sedative effect, like other benzodiazepines, and this effect long outlasts the anticonvulsant activity. Respiratory depression occurs, especially in the presence of barbiturates. Bradycardia and hypotension also complicate therapy.

Diazepam is indicated only as long as active seizures are continuing. A newer benzodiazepine, lorazepam, may be more effective than diazepam. Studies suggest that it causes less cardiorespiratory depression and has a longer duration of action (Homan and Walker, 1983).

When it appears that the attacks have temporarily ceased, or if the patient is having status epilepticus with prolonged stuporous periods between attacks, intravenous injection of phenytoin should be started immediately (Browne, 1978; Cloyd et al., 1980; Delgado-Escueta et al., 1982). In patients who are having status epilepticus with prolonged periods between attacks (sometimes called 'serial seizures') diazepam may thus be avoided entirely. The patient's already depressed consciousness will not, thereby, be further depressed by a sedative antiepileptic drug. Intravenous administration of phenytoin requires special precautions (principle 85). Phenytoin has the outstanding advantage of being nonsedative in a setting where depression of consciousness may greatly decrease the opportunity to obtain information from the neurologic examination, information that may be of great value in determining the etiology of the status episode.

If the patient does not respond to diazepam and phenytoin, phenobarbital should be given intravenously. Doses as high as 18 mg/kg — 1,000 to 1,500 mg in adults — may be required. Respiratory depression and hypotension are common, especially at high doses, and endotracheal intubation should usually be accomplished at or before this step in therapy.

Some patients simply do not respond to intravenous doses of diazepam, phenytoin, or phenobarbital, and other drugs such as paraldehyde or lidocaine may be needed. Paraldehyde can be given rectally, 5 to 10 ml in two volumes of mineral oil; it can also be given intramuscularly, 5 to 10 ml, or intravenously, 5 to 10 ml, diluted in 50 ml of normal saline (R. Simon, personal communication). Paraldehyde can cause metabolic acidosis, pulmonary hemorrhage, and cardiovascular depression. It decomposes with storage. Alternatively, lidocaine can be given as a 100-mg bolus intravenously, followed by an intravenous drip at 1 to 2 mg/min.

Although paraldehyde and lidocaine are occasionally effective, many physicians prefer to move directly to general anesthesia if phenytoin and phenobarbital fail to control the attacks. General anesthesia stops brain function, and treatment of status epilepticus may occasionally require its use. Anesthesia is usually maintained for several hours.

85. Intravenous administration of phenytoin requires precautions

The intravenous use of phenytoin has been increasing, either to achieve a loading dose or to treat status epilepticus. This increased use is appropriate, but certain measures are indicated to ensure that cardiac function is not endangered:

1. *Do not exceed a 50-mg/min infusion rate.* Administration at 25-mg/min is an excellent way to decrease the likelihood of acute

toxicity even further. However, some experienced neurologists have used a 100 mg/min infusion rate without difficulty, suggesting that the margin of safety in many patients is quite large. The clinical setting and the experience of the physician should obviously be considered when determining the infusion rate. The risk is generally much higher in the older patient than in the younger one. Patients with a history of cardiac arrhythmias, hypotension, or compromised pulmonary function should be closely monitored (Cloyd et al., 1980).

2. *Use a cardiac monitor.* Since cardiac arrhythmias from either phenytoin or the vehicle, propylene glycol (Louis et al., 1967), are the most likely form of acute toxicity, monitoring of the cardiac rhythm is indicated and will help provide early warning of cardiotoxicity.

3. *Take the blood pressure every 2 to 4 min during the infusion.* Acute hypotension is an indication to slow or discontinue the infusion.

4. *Direct intravenous injection is greatly preferable to slower infusion by intravenous drip.* When mixed with intravenous solutions, phenytoin precipitates as the pH is lowered during the dilution process. Never mix phenytoin with glucose-containing solutions, as precipitation is much more rapid and extensive. The use of 'piggyback' administration of phenytoin is somewhat controversial. In this method, phenytoin is mixed with 50 to 100 ml of physiologic saline for intravenous drip. The slower administration of a drip may be safer from the standpoint of cardiac toxicity, but microcrystallization occurs, even in physiologic saline, within 30 min (Raskin and Fishman, 1976). Some investigators recommend a filter (0.22 or 0.45 μm) to trap these crystals (Cloyd et al., 1980). It seems unlikely that small crystals would remain in that state for more than an instant after contacting plasma albumin, which binds phenytoin avidly (Porter and Layzer, 1975), and the danger therefore appears to be small. Nevertheless, the introduction of particulate material, potentially embolic, into the bloodstream is of theoretical clinical importance at the very least. A new buffered formulation of phenytoin for intravenous drip use will soon be available. Its stability in solution will obviate the current precipitation problems.

5. *Aim for a total dose of at least 13 mg/kg.* One of the most important errors is to give an inadequate dose and then to conclude prematurely that the drug is ineffective. Some investigators recommend 18 mg/kg (Cloyd et al., 1980). In status epilepticus, the chief concerns with intravenously administered phenytoin are the cardiotoxic symptoms during the acute period of administration, rather than the resultant toxicity of giving an excessive total dose. The latter can be alleviated by a reduction in dose after the acute period, and in most patients in whom intravenous administration of phenytoin is indicated, temporary dose-related ataxia will not be a problem since they are

likely to be bedfast. Monitoring plasma phenytoin levels can be extremely useful throughout the entire process of therapy and can help to indicate when maintenance therapy should be instituted. Usually, such therapy should begin about 12 hr after the loading dose has been given.

Finally, for patients who are awake and who can take oral medication, oral administration of phenytoin is an effective way to give a loading dose. With oral administration, therapeutic levels can be reached within a few hours — not fast enough for the treatment of status epilepticus, but sufficient for many non-urgent problems.

CHAPTER THIRTEEN

Therapy: The Role of Sedative Antiepileptic Drugs

86. Avoid the use of barbiturates and benzodiazepines whenever possible.

Although all long-term antiepileptic medication is subject to scrutiny for its subtle effects on cognition and memory, and although phenytoin, for example, appears to some deleterious effect on mental function, most neurologists agree that the worst offenders in this regard are the barbiturates and the benzodiazepines, which are still considered by many to be essential for the treatment of epilepsy.

Evidence for the direct deleterious effects of barbiturates on general intelligence, perceptual motor tests, memory, performance tests, and behavior has been reviewed in a study of the removal of sedative-hypnotic antiepileptic drugs (Theodore and Porter, 1983a). In a study by Vining et al. (1982), 21 children with epilepsy were given, in a double-blind crossover design, either phenobarbital or valproate. Therapeutic plasma levels of each drug were maintained for 6 months. Deleterious effects on Wechsler Intelligence Scale results and other performance test scores during phenobarbital administration documented the interference in mental function caused by phenobarbital as compared with a nonsedative antiepileptic drug. Theodore and Porter (1983a) removed all sedative antiepileptic drugs from 78 patients with severe epilepsy. No patient was left on a barbiturate, desoxybarbiturate, benzodiazepine, or even bromide. The regimens were altered to include only appropriate nonsedative drugs at appropriate doses. Seizure frequency actually improved in some patients, and only one patient was worse. Toxicity was decreased in 46 patients (59%), with decreases noted in diplopia, ataxia, daytime sleepiness, and behavior problems. This study shows that sedative antiepileptic drugs are not necessary for optimal seizure control, even in severely affected patients, and that the removal of such drugs from the regimen may decrease medication toxicity.

The toxic effects of clonazepam are similar to and at least as severe as those of phenobarbital. Most common are drowsiness, ataxia, and behavioral and personality changes (Dreifuss and Sato, 1982). Respiratory tract secretions may also increase. In a study of clonazepam in 37 patients with absence seizures, 10 could not complete the study because of side effects of the drug

Table 86.1. Toxicity of clonazepam in 37 patients with absence seizures

Side effect	No. of patients
Drowsiness	21
Ataxia	16
Hyperactivity	12
Weight gain	11
Nystagmus	9
Personality change	7
Increased seizures	6
Change in seizure type	3
Leukopenia	1

From Dreifuss and Sato (1982).

(Table 86.1). Nitrazepam is less potent and may be slightly less toxic, but the reported side effects are fundamentally the same as for clonazepam (Baruzzi et al., 1982).

In summary, there is little evidence that the current antiepileptic drug regimen, for most seizure types, is improved by the addition of barbiturates or benzodiazepines. There is considerable evidence that long-term use of these sedative agents has a deleterious effect. These drugs can be withdrawn, even in outpatients (principle 89). Following sedative drug withdrawal, most adults are more alert, and most children have improved behavior.

87. Many antiepileptic barbiturates are metabolized to phenobarbital.

Anecdotal reports suggest that some antiepileptic barbiturates are preferable to others. Usually, this favoring of one barbiturate over another is based on an opinion that the favored drug has fewer side effects (especially sedation or hyperactivity) or that these side effects are somewhat less severe. All doctors who treat epileptic patients have seen occasional patients in whom the decreased toxicity of one barbiturate over another seemed convincing.

Unfortunately, the hypothesis that one barbiturate is less toxic than another is especially hard to test because the majority of such drugs (except phenobarbital itself) have an active metabolite, usually phenobarbital. Even if one were inclined to test clinically one drug against another, it would never be possible to eliminate the problem of a common, active metabolite with known toxic side effects. The common and uncommon barbiturates used in the United States for seizure control are shown in Table 87.1.

Phenobarbital has no known active metabolites; the principal metabolite is p-hydroxyphenobarbital. Primidone (a desoxybarbiturate) is more complex. As the parent compound, it has activity comparable to that of

Table 87.1.   Antiepileptic barbiturates used in the United States

Drug	Active metabolite
Phenobarbital	None known
Primidone	Phenobarbital, phenylethylmalonamide
Mephobarbital	Phenobarbital
Metharbital	Barbital
Barbital	None known
Eterobarb (experimental in U.S.)	Phenobarbital

phenobarbital, but it is also converted to phenobarbital and phenylethylmalonamide. The latter appears to have but little antiepileptic effect (Bourgeois et al., 1982). The plasma phenobarbital level produced by primidone is variable; it may equal the primidone level, or more commonly (and especially in the presence of other drugs), be two or three times as high.

Mephobarbital is converted to phenobarbital to the extent that most patients have about 20 times more phenobarbital in their plasma than they have of the parent compound (Kupferberg and Longacre-Shaw, 1979). Metharbital is changed to barbital, which in turn is apparently excreted unchanged (Maynert, 1972). Little information is available on the efficacy of this drug or its metabolite. Eterobarb, or dimethoxymethylphenobarbital, is rapidly metabolized by the liver, and although minor metabolites have been identified, the antiepileptic action of the drug can be completely explained by its conversion to phenobarbital (Goldberg, 1982).

88. Primidone and phenobarbital should not be used together.

If the use of barbiturates is discouraged (principle 86), then the use of two sedative drugs simultaneously seems especially unwarranted. With the combination of primidone and phenobarbital, the likelihood of improved seizure control is greatly outweighed by the potential for toxicity. Since primidone is rapidly converted in large part to phenobarbital, the effect is one of adding a metabolite when both phenobarbital and primidone are prescribed. It is theoretically possible, of course, to accomplish such a regimen with careful monitoring of plasma levels of both drugs, but only in the most unusual circumstances is this ever warranted. The addition of phenobarbital to primidone often causes a remarkably high level of phenobarbital, with additional sedative and behavioral toxicity. When primidone is combined with phenytoin, enhancement of phenobarbital levels also occurs (Porro et al., 1982).

If phenobarbital must be used, its therapeutic plasma levels range from 15 to 40 μg/ml (Porter and Penry, 1980). Therapeutic primidone levels are usually in the range of 6 to 15 μg/ml. Primidone should be started at low doses and gradually increased. It is only marginally possible to obtain maximal efficacy with these drugs by increasing their plasma levels to the toxic range, as many patients have subtle toxic effects in the therapeutic range.

89. Barbiturates and benzodiazepines can be withdrawn in outpatients.

When the judgment has been made that a patient may profit from fewer antiepileptic drugs, or when the patient is taking a barbiturate, desoxybarbiturate, or benzodiazepine, it is reasonable to consider a decrease in the sedative medications. The manner in which this can be accomplished is especially dependent on the propensity of the patient to have generalized tonic-clonic seizures. A patient with absence attacks only, and no history of generalized tonic-clonic seizures, may have drugs withdrawn with relative safety. Even if a generalized tonic-clonic seizure occurs, the likelihood of status epilepticus is remote, especially if the patient is simultaneously being treated with valproate. In a patient with frequent complex partial seizures, with secondary generalized tonic-clonic seizures every month or two, the precautions must be much more vigorous. Clearly, it is necessary to protect the patient with appropriate drugs against the occurrence of generalized tonic-clonic seizures during the withdrawal period. The most effective regimen, especially for severely affected patients, is a combination of phenytoin and carbamazepine in maximally tolerated doses, which usually means trough plasma levels of approximately 18 to 20 μg/ml for phenytoin and 6 to 7 μg/ml for carbamazepine. Status epilepticus is uncommon in patients so protected during the withdrawal period, *providing* that the withdrawal period is reasonably long.

The rate of withdrawal is an important aspect of antiepileptic drug discontinuation. Regardless of the long half-life of both barbiturates and benzodiazepines, a prolonged withdrawal period, with careful monitoring and frequent follow-up is the safest way of preventing serious problems. Phenobarbital withdrawal problems are greatest at the lower end of the therapeutic range; few problems are usually encountered, for example, in dropping the plasma phenobarbital level from 60 to 30 μg/ml, but generalized tonic-clonic attacks may occur as the level falls below 15 μg/ml. Antiepileptic drug doses should be decreased over many weeks, especially if barbiturates and benzodiazepines are being withdrawn.

It is also important to distinguish between withdrawal seizures and seizures occurring because of inadequate medication. A common error in the attempt to remove barbiturates occurs when the patient's seizures temporarily worsen and the physician assumes that the worsening indicates a *need* for the barbiturate rather than a withdrawal phenomenon. The result is continuation of a sedative antiepileptic drug that may not be needed. In many patients it is important to try to 'weather the storm' of withdrawal; the gains may be well worth the effort.

Theodore and Porter (1983b) successfully withdrew all sedative-hypnotic

Table 89.1. Mean doses and plasma levels of antiepileptic drugs taken by 38 outpatients

	Before Withdrawal			After Withdrawal	
	Dose (mg/day)	Plasma level (μg/ml)		Dose (mg/day)	Plasma level (μg/ml)
Primidone	808	7.2		0	0
Phenobarbital	115	33.2		0	0
Clonazepam	3	—		0	0
Phenytoin	309	13.5		363	18.2
Carbamazepine	1,062	4.0		1,144	6.5

From Theodore and Porter (1983b).

drugs from 38 outpatients referred for intractable seizures. The patients ranged from 5 to 63 years of age. Withdrawal of the drugs took place over an average of 12 weeks in each patient. Primidone was the most commonly prescribed barbiturate and clonazepam the most common benzodiazepine. Withdrawal was generally well tolerated, with 11 patients reporting a transient increase in seizure frequency during the withdrawal period. Sedative-hypnotic drugs were temporarily restarted in three patients, one of whom was hospitalized for 2 days. Status epilepticus did not occur. At follow-up, averaging 17 months after drug withdrawal, 32 of the patients showed improvement in either seizure frequency or medication toxicity, or both. Six patients were unchanged, but no patient was worse. Table 89.1 shows the mean doses and plasma levels of the patients' drugs before and after withdrawal of the first three. Noteworthy is the increase in the mean plasma phenytoin level from 13.5 to 18.2 μg/ml and in the mean carbamazepine level from 4.0 to 6.5 µg/ml. The largest increases in plasma levels of phenytoin and carbamazepine were accomplished early in the withdrawal period to minimize withdrawal seizures.

Another difficult problem is the discontinuation of all medication in patients who have been seizure free for some time. The heterogeneity of epilepsy makes such decisions difficult, but most patients should have a gradual discontinuation of medications, especially if more than one drug is being used, after 3 or 4 years without seizures. In a study of 68 children, Emerson et al. (1981) concluded that four seizure-free years is an appropriate waiting period if the child had not had many seizures and if the EEG is not prominently abnormal. Drugs were successfully withdrawn from more than two-thirds of the patients without seizure recurrence.

CHAPTER FOURTEEN

Therapy: The Role of Surgery in Epilepsy

90. Surgical therapy should be considered for medically intractable partial seizures.

The number of epileptic patients whose attacks remain uncontrolled by current forms of treatment is quite large and probably extends to at least 25% of all epileptic patients. In the United States, for example, approximately 200,000 persons have seizures more than once a month (Commission, 1978), and the number of patients with uncontrolled partial seizures is estimated to be 360,000 (Ward, 1983). Many of these patients could benefit from improved medical therapy, including advanced clinical pharmacologic techniques, but the majority will not become seizure free (Porter et al, 1977). All of these patients deserve consideration for surgical therapy, as the localized nature of the causal lesion is the first and most important criterion for consideration. Such consideration is important even though many will be eventually rejected on various criteria (principle 91).

Ward (1983) has estimated that at least 15% of the 360,000 patients with uncontrolled partial seizures are candidates for surgery—54,000 candidates, yet the number of operations for epilepsy in the United States is probably not much more than 100 a year. The underutilization of surgical therapy for epilepsy is presumably related to an assumption that medical therapy is more effective than it actually is, the need for expensive and dedicated teams to evaluate patients and to perform appropriate surgical procedures, and inadequate education of the primary care physician about the value of surgical therapy (Ward, 1983).

In summary, patients with intractable partial seizures should be considered as possible surgical candidates if they are unresponsive to available medications. These patients should be referred to specialized epilepsy centers.

91. The selection of patients for surgical intervention is constantly being reevaluated.

The patient with intractable complex partial seizures and a clear-cut unilateral temporal lobe focus is the ideal candidate for surgical intervention.

113

A series of decisions must be made for each surgical therapy candidate. These decisions are discussed below in the approximate order of their consideration; the approach is basically taken from Rasmussen (1975).

1. *Is the patient's epilepsy medically intractable?* The vast majority of epileptic patients considered for surgical therapy will have partial seizures. The use of maximally tolerated doses of both phenytoin and carbamazepine (principle 63) is the most reasonable approach to establish whether medical therapy will be adequate. The addition of primidone or other sedative drug to such a regimen is unlikely to improve seizure control and will add toxicity. Some investigators feel that other drugs should, nevertheless, be tried for completeness of effort.

   After the patient is receiving a maximally tolerated regimen of antiepileptic drugs, the significance of the seizures and their frequency must be evaluated in terms of the resulting disability. As noted by Rasmussen (1975), some patients can easily tolerate brief or nocturnal seizures without noticeable interference with daily activities. In others, even brief seizures may jeopardize a job or prevent driving a car. In patients who are on sedative-hypnotic drugs, the incapacity caused by the side effects of the medication must also be considered. The intractability of the seizures should be prolonged, that is, spontaneous improvement of the disorder should clearly be unlikely before surgical therapy is considered.

2. *Does the patient really want the operation?* The patient must be motivated to undergo the testing necessary to establish eligibility for surgical therapy and to localize the lesion, and finally the patient must be willing to cooperate with the surgical procedure itself. The prolonged process and the associated discomfort and risks should be carefully explained to the patient. The motivation should not come primarily from the family or from the physician (Rasmussen, 1975).

3. *How well localized is the epileptogenic lesion?* Many criteria can be applied to localization of the lesion, which must be somewhat discrete and not located in or closely adjacent to vital structures, such as the speech area. Clinical clues come directly from the history of the seizures; auras need to be evaluated, aphasia or other localizing symptoms must be sought, and the onset of the attack should be determined in detail. Neuropsychologic studies will add to the data on localization.

   Electroencephalographic data are critical in the effort to localize the lesion. Initial studies are routine, but the addition of more specialized efforts include simultaneous video and EEG recordings, the use of sphenoidal leads, and the intracarotid sodium amytal test. The need for invasive studies to obtain electrographic evidence of the seizure focus is controversial and evolving. Some investigators routinely implant depth electrodes to assure maximal information. Others use depth electrodes sparingly and prefer subdural strip electrodes when scalp recordings do not give definitive results. Direct cortical recording during the operation to confirm and further define the lesion is now nearly routine.

Specialized brain imaging techniques, especially PET and NMR, have great potential for altering the approach to selection of surgical candidates and for defining surgical lesions (principle 100).

For those patients with temporal lobe lesions who undergo cortical excision, the results are quite promising. In 653 patients with a median follow-up of 11 years, Rasmussen (1975) reported that 71% either had become seizure free or had a marked reduction in frequency of attacks. The current morbidity and mortality rates of the excisional procedures are quite low.

Finally, only minimal progress is being made in surgical approaches to nonlocalized lesions. Notable among the failures is the cerebellar stimulator, which was initially received enthusiastically, but in a double-blind study (Van Buren et al., 1978) was shown to be ineffective. Splitting of the corpus callosum remains experimental; the data on its clinical utility are inconclusive and largely anecdotal.

CHAPTER FIFTEEN

Therapy: Pregnancy and Epilepsy

92. Reevaluate all antiepileptic drugs used in pregnant epileptic patients.

One of the most controversial subjects related to epilepsy is the proper management of pregnant epileptic patients and their offspring. In this chapter, the maternal and fetal concerns are arbitrarily separated; the maternal issues are addressed below, and the fetal issues in principle 93.

1. *Does pregnancy cause epilepsy?* Only an occasional case report confirms the occurrence of seizures limited to pregnancy (Teare, 1980). Ordinarily, pregnancy is not considered a cause of epilepsy except as a complication of other neurologic insults, such as cerebral sinus thrombosis.

2. *Does pregnancy worsen epilepsy?* Available data suggest that about half the patients with epilepsy who become pregnant will have no change in their seizure frequency. The remaining half is roughly divided between those who do better and those who do worse (Schmidt, 1981). The chief factors in worsening of seizure frequency during pregnancy seem to be related to poor compliance and altered absorption or metabolism of drugs.

3. *Does eclampsia cause epilepsy?* Although epileptic seizures may occur during severe eclampsia, there is little evidence that the seizures will persist after delivery and recovery from the metabolic disturbances.

4. *Does status epilepticus occur more frequently during pregnancy?* Fortunately, there does not appear to be an increased incidence of status epilepticus during pregnancy (Schmidt, 1981). Obviously, however, the prevention of generalized tonic-clonic status is of great importance.

5. *How will pregnancy change the pharmacological action of antiepileptic drugs?* Changes may not occur at all or they may involve alterations in absorption, plasma protein binding, metabolism, and volume of distribution. If a change occurs, it is usually a fall in plasma drug levels, which return to normal after delivery. The only sure way to maintain seizure control is to monitor the plasma drug levels more frequently

Table 92.1. Recommendations for managing the pregnant epileptic patient.

---

   1. Establish a drug regimen that
        a. gives optimal seizure control
        b. has few side effects
        c. requires the least number of drugs
        d. does not include trimethadione or valproate
   2. Make few major changes in the regimen, but
        a. see the patient monthly
        b. determine plasma drug levels at each visit
        c. change the regimen only if control worsens considerably
   3. Avoid status epilepticus by
        a. maintaining therapeutic plasma drug levels
        b. emphasizing patient compliance
   4. Avoid toxicity after delivery by
        a. decreasing antiepileptic drug doses slightly
        b. following plasma drug levels closely for 2 to 3 weeks

---

Modified from Montouris et al. (1979).

during pregnancy.

6. *Are bleeding tendencies altered by antiepileptic drug therapy?* Some evidence suggests that bleeding tendencies may be increased in neonates born to mothers taking antiepileptic drugs (principle 93).

7. *How common are compliance problems during pregnancy?* According to Schmidt (1981), poor compliance is one of the most likely causes of increased seizures during pregnancy. Patients have problems with compliance under the best of circumstances, but with the added stress of possible teratogenic effects of the antiepileptic drugs, many patients take their drugs even less compulsively.

8. *In general, what should be the physician's plan for the pregnant epileptic patient?* Overall, the physician should not change his fundamental approach to the treatment of seizures, but should monitor the patient more closely. Specific recommendations are given in Table 92.1.

93. Fetal abnormalities are slightly more frequent if the mother has epilepsy.

The issues regarding the fetus in the pregnant epileptic patient are controversial; many answers are not available to some of the most important questions. The principal issues concerning the fetus are as follows:

1. *Is epilepsy inherited?* Some generalized seizures appear, in some families, to be inherited. Examples are absence seizures and primary generalized tonic-clonic seizures. In most cases of epilepsy, however, inheritance does not appear to be implicated; this is especially true for partial seizures. Bearing children is not to be condemned *a priori* in patients with epilepsy; only infrequently will there be sufficient genetic evidence to discourage pregnancy. Presumably, the father's contribution to inheritance of epilepsy is as great as the mother's. The influence

of hereditary factors on fetal abnormalities is obscure and difficult to separate from the possible effects of antiepileptic drugs.

2. *Do antiepileptic drugs cause fetal abnormalities?* The drugs used for epilepsy probably cause abnormalities of the fetus in a small number of pregnancies. The abnormalities are often minor; a few are severe. Of the abnormalities associated with anitepileptic drugs, the fetal hydantoin syndrome of phenytoin (Table 93.1) has been best described. However, these abnormalities may also be observed with the use of other antiepileptic drugs. The diones, trimethadione and paramethadione, may be associated with a higher incidence of abnormalities than some other drugs and should be avoided. Recent studies on valproate suggest an increased incidence of spina bifida (Bjerkedal et al., 1982), an observation which, though it requires further investigation, must be strongly considered in the choice of drugs during pregnancy.

3. *Which is more likely to cause malformations—heredity or antiepileptic drugs?* No one knows the answer to this question. Although epileptic women who are not treated with antiepileptic drugs during pregnancy apparently have a lower incidence of fetal abnormalities than those who take medications (Hanson and Buehler, 1982), it is possible that those who need medication also have increased hereditary factors. There is little evidence that maternal seizures, in themselves, contribute to an increased frequency of fetal malformations.

4. *Do antiepileptic drugs have a direct toxic effect on the fetus?* All antiepileptic drugs are transferred to the fetus across the placenta. Several short- and long-term effects of these drugs on the fetus have been suggested. Neonatal depression has been described, but is rarely severe and only occurs if the mother has received sedative antiepileptic

Table 93.1.   Fetal hydantoin syndrome: most common abnormalities in five children

1. Growth and Performance
   a.   Motor or mental deficiency
   b.   Microcephaly
   c.   Postnatal growth deficiency

2. Craniofacial
   a.   Short nose with low nasal bridge
   b.   Hypertelorism
   c.   Low-set or abnormal ears
   d.   Short or webbed neck

3. Limb
   a.   Hypoplasia of nails and distal phalanges
   b.   Finger-like thumb

From Hanson and Smith (1975).

drugs. Frank withdrawal symptoms in the neonate are exceedingly uncommon. The long-term effect of these drugs on brain and body development is unknown, although numerous experimental studies suggest that they may have deleterious effects. Antiepileptic drugs are transferred in breast milk to the child. Although few complications of such transfer have been described, some recommend reduced breast feeding (Kaneko et al., 1981). Newborns apparently do not develop biochemical signs of osteomalacia from antiepileptic drugs (Christiansen et al., 1980). Some have observed an increase in stillbirths, neonatal mortality, and neonatal jaundice in children of epileptic mothers or fathers (Janz and Beck-Mannagetta, 1981).

5. *What is the overall risk of fetal abnormalities in children born to epileptic parents?* Overall, a twofold or threefold increase in the risk of fetal abnormalities is the current consensus. If the usual rate of abnormalities is considered to be 2%, then the likelihood may be 4% to 6% in such children. Parents should be counseled regarding this increased overall risk.

6. *How should the newborn be managed?* Each newborn of a mother taking antiepileptic drugs should receive 1 mg of vitamin K (phytonadione) immediately after birth. Clotting factors should be monitored every 2 to 4 hr, and additional vitamin K should be administered until these factors are normal (Montouris et al., 1979).

CHAPTER SIXTEEN

Psychosocial Aspects of Epilepsy

94. Psychiatric disorders in patients with epilepsy should be treated in the usual manner.

Patients with epilepsy appear to have an increased incidence of psychiatric disorders, but the disorders are the same as those affecting other people. They include both neuroses, such as depression or personality disorders, and psychoses. Controversy about the causes of such disorders abounds, and concerns, for example, the contribution of temporal lobe abnormalities to psychoses or specific personality traits. According to Pond (1981), 'the relationship between type of personality change and type of epilepsy is...complex and few figures are available, even to confirm or deny the special psychological disorders associated with temporal lobe epilepsy.' The diagnosis and treatment of psychiatric disorders in epileptic patients does not differ greatly from that of other psychiatric patients who do not have epilepsy. The chief difficulty, as noted by Rodin (1975), is in the interaction of the neurologist and the psychiatrist, who must continuously communicate with each other if the patient's various symptoms are to be properly managed. Having a consultant psychiatrist who understands epilepsy is of equal importance to having a neurologist sensitive to psychiatric symptoms.

The use of drugs in the treatment of psychiatric disease in epileptic patients is not as complex as might be thought, and necessary psychotropic drugs should not be withheld from these patients. First, the use of nonsedative regimens (principle 86) will provide a significant first step toward decreasing negative effects on the psyche, especially depression. Second, carbamazepine is useful in patients with mania (Post and Cutler, 1979) and perhaps depression as well. Some evidence suggests that some newer antidepressants may not decrease seizure threshold (Trimble, 1981). The tricyclic antidepressants, however, are only infrequently associated with increased seizures, and although precautions are necessary, these drugs should be used whenever they are needed. The same is true for the phenothiazines (Toone, 1981), which can be given to patients already on antiepileptic drugs without seizure exacerbation (Rodin, 1975). A complete review of the psychiatric problems in epilepsy is available (Reynolds and Trimble, 1981).

95. Persons with epilepsy are more limited by the fearful reactions of others than by the seizures themselves.

In many areas of social adaptation, in which epileptic patients might be expected to function normally, avenues are often cut off because of misunderstandings that generate inappropriate fears about people with epilepsy. A comprehensive analysis of the problem is beyond the scope of this book, but one example, that of employment, will serve to illustrate the problem.

The rate of unemployment is twice as high among people with epilepsy as the national average. Although the majority of patients with epilepsy are medically restored to a functional degree, they are often denied the opportunity to work because of the fears of the potential employer. The first of the fears to allay is the employer's fear of increased cost. In the United States, many employers are afraid that their contribution to workman's compensation will increase if they hire a person with epilepsy. Because of the way in which rates under workman's compensation are calculated, however, the rates do not increase if a person with epilepsy is hired, because the underwriting process is performed without reference to the health of the employee (Eilers and Melone, undated). Employees can only increase the employer's premiums if they increase the average frequency or severity of losses. Since there is a considerable consensus that persons with epilepsy incur no more injuries than other employees (Eilers and Melone, undated), the actual risk of increased cost is exceedingly small.

The employer is responsible for hiring an individual who would not have a high likelihood of injury because of the nature of the job itself. Persons with epilepsy, therefore, are often appropriately denied jobs near moving machinery or in high places. The employer must be satisfied that the particular job does not pose an unexpectedly high risk for that particular employee. The risks to the employer can be minimized if the following characteristics are considered in relation to the proposed job (Commission, 1978). Most jobs can bè performed by persons whose epilepsy is represented at the top of the following list; a smaller but fair number of jobs can be performed even by persons whose seizures are at the bottom of the list:

1. The attacks are under complete control.
2. The attacks occur with predictable time of occurrence in relation to hours of work—at night, for example.
3. The attacks occur without loss of consciousness or loss of voluntary control.
4. The attacks are preceded by at least 30 sec of warning prior to unconsciousness or loss of voluntary control.
5. The attacks are without loss of consciousness but with loss of voluntary control.
6. The attacks are associated with loss of consciousness but not with falling.

7. The attacks are associated with loss of consciousness and automatic behavior.
8. The attacks are characterized by falling without warning.

In any case, the capabilities of each individual should be assessed and placement should first be based on the individual's ability rather than on his disability.

96. Persons with epilepsy require a comprehensive approach to their medical and social needs.

As with other complex disorders, the difficulty of managing the person with epilepsy does not end with medical care delivery; it extends to the social adaptation and, if necessary, rehabilitation of the affected person. In general, ascending levels of medical and psychosocial care delivery should be available to the person with epilepsy. The various levels are determined by the severity of the problems.

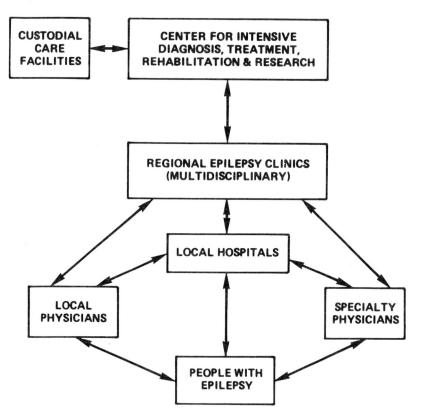

Fig. 96.1. The pyramidal structure of care for patients with epilepsy in the United States (see text). (From Cereghino et al., 1980)

The effort to deliver comprehensive medical and social care to the person with epilepsy is world-wide. In Kenya, for example, a large number of local dispensaries handle the usual patient. If the problem is more complex, the patient is referred to one of 400 Health Centers, where more experienced health care technicians are available. If further evaluation or treatment is required, the patient is sent to one of the more than 50 District Hospitals, which have full medical and surgical services. For most patients, the ultimate referral center is one of seven Provincial Hospitals, but the top of the pyramid is the National Hospital in Nairobi (Tower, 1978).

A similar structure exists in the United States (Fig. 96.1). Persons with epilepsy deal directly with their personal physician or with a specialty physician, and in some cases (especially those without health insurance), with a local hospital. In the ideal setting, the more difficult patients are referred to a regional clinic that specializes in epilepsy; many university hospitals serve this function quite well. Finally, the most difficult patients are referred to a comprehensive center for intensive diagnosis and treatment of their epilepsy and for evaluation and assistance with their psychosocial needs. The team at such centers is usually composed of professionals in neurology, neurosurgery, psychiatry, psychology, electroencephalography, social work, and rehabilitation counseling (Rodin, 1975). Such centers are often conducting clinical investigations and may have appropriate research protocols for voluntary participation. Following intensive evaluation at the comprehensive center, a few patients may require long-term custodial care, but their occasional reevaluation should be assured (Cereghino et al., 1980).

Many countries offer ultimate care in a National Epilepsy Center. Such centers deal with the most difficult patients, but are also able to attract highly qualified, dedicated professional staffs. They often combine the very best in intensive diagnosis and treatment, vocational rehabilitation, and research. Successful rehabilitation of the patients is the matter of greatest concern, and their return to society usually represents a considerable accomplishment.

97. The degree of social adaptation in work, school, and recreation is the final criterion for health care delivery to the patient with epilepsy.

Although the doctor is often the most effective advocate for the psychosocial well-being of the patient with epilepsy, he sometimes abdicates this responsibility. Listed below are some areas of special concern that have a direct impact on the opportunities available to persons with epilepsy:

1. *Prevention*: The physician has long been an advocate for prevention of disease, but the prevention of epilepsy requires special emphasis on perinatal care, childhood infections, and, most importantly, head injury. The number of new cases of epilepsy in England caused by head injury is 5,000 annually; in the United States, the number is probably about 20,000 new cases each year. Most head injuries are from motor vehicle accidents. There is strong evidence that lower

speed limits (such as the 55-mph limit in the United States), helmet laws for motorcyclists, restraint systems (such as belts or air bags), and vigorous prosecution of intoxicated drivers will contribute greatly to a decreased incidence of posttraumatic epilepsy.

2. *Education*: During the schoolyears, the child with epilepsy requires understanding, but should participate in as many normal activities as possible. Teachers should be well-informed about epilepsy; their attitude is critical. Severely affected children deserve special classes and should be treated in a manner appropriate to their disability. For adults, vocational training is the only way in which many will become self-sufficient.

3. *Mental health*: Although the primary care physician or neurologist may not feel competent to manage the occasional psychiatric problems of epileptic patients, an effective referral pattern must be established by each doctor, with special attention to patients who find psychiatric care difficult to obtain for financial or other reasons. The fundamental pharmacologic approach to these patients is discussed in principle 94.

4. *Counseling*: The doctor should be available for counseling of his patients, but should also be aware of the community counseling services.

5. *Employment*: This most difficult problem is discussed in principle 95.

6. *Insurance*: Persons with epilepsy often have great difficulties in obtaining insurance of all types, including life, health, and automobile insurance. Often the premiums are high, and for the unemployed person, not within financial reach.

7. *Driving*: More realistic laws are gradually being adopted to allow persons with a history of epileptic seizures to drive. Patients must be seizure free for 2 years in the United Kingdom but usually only for 1 year in the United States, depending on the various state laws. In the United Kingdom, patients who suffer only nocturnal attacks may drive after a 3-year period.

There is no adequate answer for the patient who has been seizure free, has obtained a license to drive, and who wishes to consider withdrawal of antiepileptic drugs. A single seizure, with resultant loss of the driver's license, may jeopardize the patient's job and financial well-being. Many patients choose to continue long-term drug therapy, risking medication toxicity instead of risking loss of the driver's license. Withdrawal of antiepileptic drugs is discussed in detail in principle 89.

8. *Recreational needs*: Although a few sports are unreasonably danger-ous for many persons with epilepsy, such as unsupervised swimming or activities associated with dangerous heights, the doctor should usually advocate vigorous recreational activity. Such activities are easily inhibited by fears of rejection or 'being different,' especially in

children. Except in the most unusual cases, worsening of the epilepsy does not occur during exercise, and most patients profit from strong encouragement.

9. *Lay organizations*: Strong support of lay organizations that are concerned with epilepsy will result in a gradual improvement of these psychosocial problems. Physicians can be especially effective, not so much in direct leadership, but in support of lay persons who are attempting to improve the plight of people with epilepsy.

CHAPTER SEVENTEEN

The Future: Research Considerations

98. We need to know more about the basic mechanisms of the epilepsies and of antiepileptic drugs.

Our understanding of the basic mechanisms of the epilepsies is quite limited, and much more work is needed for basic knowledge to have a direct impact on the diagnosis and therapy of seizures. To show just a glimpse of the kinds of studies being performed, brief discussions of two different mechanisms follow; one is a basic understanding of the epileptic process in partial epilepsy, and the other is a postulated mechanism of action of an antiepileptic drug.

In experimental focal epilepsy, the fundamental alteration of the neuron's membrane potential is called the paroxysmal depolarization shift (PDS), discovered almost two decades ago. During the PDS (Fig. 98.1), intracellular recordings show a sudden change in the usual membrane potential, with a high-amplitude, prolonged depolarization with superimposed high-frequency spikes. Extracellular recordings show only the spikes, and the scalp-recorded EEG shows a negative spike. The PDS is usually followed by strong afterhyperpolarization, which presumably inhibits cell firing; the scalp-recorded EEG may show a slow wave. If the afterhyperpolarization becomes less intense (for unexplained reasons), the frequency of the PDS's will increase, leading to a seizure. During the tonic portion of the seizure, the membrane is maintained in a depolarized state (Fig. 98.1). As the afterhyperpolarizations increase again, the clonic phase ensues. When the hyperpolarization finally becomes dominant, the PDS complexes disappear, and postictal depression occurs. Although great efforts are continuing, we do not understand why a PDS occurs or why this sequence of events takes place.

The mechanism of action of one of the newest antiepileptic drugs may be related to its action on the inhibitory neurotransmitter, gamma-aminobutyric acid (GABA). In an elementary sense, if inhibitory neurotransmitters cause a decrease in neuronal firing, then perhaps the neuronal hyperactivity characteristic of epilepsy will be decreased in the presence of increased concentrations of inhibitory neurotransmitters such as GABA. Several investigators have demonstrated an increase in brain GABA levels following administration of valproate, and Ciesielski et al. (1975) showed that valproate protected audiogenic mice (i.e., mice susceptible to seizures from auditory stimuli) from seizures for 2 hr. This protection could be correlated with a rise in brain GABA apparently caused by the valproate, whose concentration in brain also increased (Fig. 98.2). Unfortunately, as with our understanding of most of the mechanisms of action of antiepileptic drugs, interpretation of these findings is clouded. For one thing, a very high dose of valproate (400 mg/kg) was needed to obtain the effect. Others have observed that valproate is not a very strong inhibitor of GABA transaminase, the major degradative enzyme and that the effect of valproate is probably not mediated by this mechanism. Furthermore, no change in GABA levels is seen when a dose of valproate necessary to block a pentylenetetrazol-induced seizure is given, although levels at the critical sites (e.g., the synapse) may theoretically increase without a noticeable increase in overall brain GABA (Kupferberg, 1980). In summary, the question remains whether valproate exerts its action via GABA, and if so, whether this action is mediated by an effect on the degradative enzyme system.

Several promising areas of investigation may provide answers to how and why epileptic seizures occur and how antiepileptic drugs inhibit and modify the

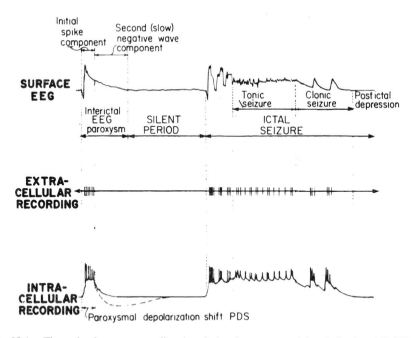

Fig. 98.1.   Three simultaneous recording sites during the paroxysmal depolarization shift (PDS): intracellular (*bottom trace*), extracellular (*middle trace*), and surface EEG (*top trace*). A single PDS on the left, accompanied by a cortical spike, is followed by hyperpolarization but not by a seizure. When afterhyperpolarization is diminished, the PDS frequency increases and a seizure occurs (see text). From Ayala et al., 1970.

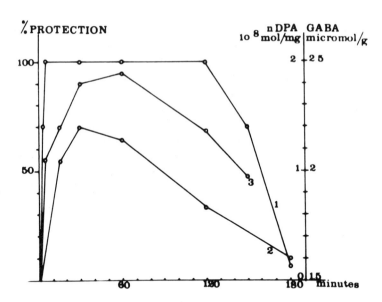

Fig 98.2. The effect of valproate on mice susceptible to audiogenic seizures (i.e., seizures induced by sudden noise). Curve 1 (*top line*) shows the percentage of seizure protection resulting from an injection of valproate, 400 mg/kg. Curve 2 (*bottom line*) shows the concentration of brain GABA, and curve 3 (*middle line*) shows the concentration of radioactive valproate in brain. See text for further discussion of this interesting correlation. (From Ciesielski et al., 1975).

attacks. Some of these are studies in neurogenetics, neuropeptides, protein phosphorylation, ionic channels and gates, kindling, cyclic nucleotides, glial interaction with neurons, and a wide variety of neurotransmitters; these important areas have recently been summarized (Delgado-Escueta et al., 1983).

99. We need better drugs for epilepsy.

The rationale for the search for new antiepileptic drugs has been expressively stated by Krall et al. (1978a): 'For many patients with epilepsy, the development of a new antiepileptic drug offers the only hope of achieving control of their seizures. For those patients whose seizures are controlled by currently available therapy, a new drug may reduce the toxic side effects they often tolerate to gain seizure control.'

In spite of the need for new antiepileptic drugs, pharmaceutical firms have been reluctant to invest in their development. The market for antiepileptic drugs is relatively small, and the research and development costs may be prohibitive as compared with the expected financial return. (Porter, 1983b).

The development of new drugs requires many separate steps, beginning with synthesis, followed by preclinical evaluation for efficacy (screening), and animal toxicity studies. The clinical studies begin, as a rule, after governmental approval of the safety of the drug. The various phases of antiepileptic drug development are shown in Fig. 99.1. The Antiepileptic Drug Development Program (ADDP) of the Epilepsy Branch, National Institute of Neurological and Communicative Disorders and Stroke, is

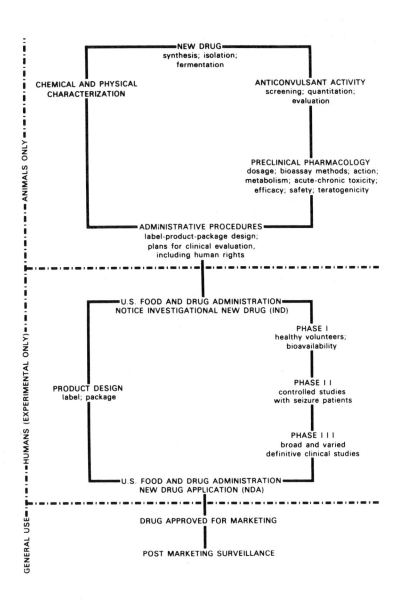

Fig. 99.1. The development of antiepileptic drugs in the United States (see text). (From Cereghino and Penry, 1982.)

concerned with all of these phases (Tower, 1978; Krall et al., 1978b; Porter, 1983b):

1. *Synthesis*: A small ADDP project allows promising academic investigators to use their ingenuity in the construction of new molecules that may have antiepileptic activity. Compounds produced by these investigators are usually sent to the antiepileptic drug screening program. Most synthesis is done independent of the ADDP project by pharmaceutical firms.

2. *Screening*: A critical part of any drug development program is the testing for efficacy in animal models, an area in which epilepsy has a considerable advantage over many other disorders. Compounds are accepted by the ADDP screening project from academicians and pharmaceutical firms all over the world. The compounds are screened in mice by the maximal electroshock seizure test (which correlates with partial seizures and generalized tonic-clonic seizures in humans), and the pentylenetetrazol seizure test (which correlates with absence seizures in humans); the rotorod toxicity test, a neurologic test of ataxia, is also performed. The compounds are further tested in rats and in other experimental models of seizures (i.e., bicuculline-, strychnine-, and picrotoxin-induced seizures). As of early 1983, the screening program had tested more than 7,000 compounds. A handful of promising potential antiepileptic drugs has emerged, and some of these have been evaluated in the next phase, the toxicology project.

3. *Toxicology*: Even though confronted with a compound that may be efficacious, pharmaceutical firms are still faced with expensive toxicity testing before the drug can be tried clinically. For this reason, a limited number of compunds are selected after screening for further study in the ADDP toxicology project. This project evaluates their safety in 90-day investigations in rats and dogs. The intent is to prove that the compound is safe enough for a definitive clinical efficacy trial.

4. *Human studies*: Human studies do not usually begin in patients, but in healthy volunteers. The studies are designed primarily to test the clinical safety of the drugs. Such studies often last less than a month and determine the range of tolerated doses. These investigations are referred to as phase I studies.

   Following the volunteer studies, patient studies begin. Pilot studies are usually followed by controlled clinical trials, which are commonly double-blind, that is, neither the patient nor the doctor knows whether the drug or a placebo is being taken. In the United States, two well-controlled clinical trials are necessary; both must demonstrate antiepileptic effectiveness. Long-term evaluation of the compound in a large number of patients follows the definitive efficacy testing. Such studies often include patients tested in earlier clinical investigations. Exposing the drug to a large number of patients helps uncover unusual reactions and provides further evidence of its effectiveness. The clinical studies in patients are often termed phase II and phase III studies.

The clinical study of epilepsy is fraught with a multitude of difficult scientific and ethical problems. Some of these problems include the study of patients with severe seizures, with partially controlled seizures, with seizures of ill-defined nature, and with multiple concomitant medical regimens. The ADDP clinical trials project is currently sponsoring several clinical trials of new and novel compounds.

Antiepileptic drug development is in a stage of expansion that allows greater and greater specificity of medication tailored to the specific seizure type. As new drugs are developed, old ones will be replaced. No regimen should be considered infinitely useful. There is always the distinct possibility of change in the light of new drugs and technological advances.

100.   New diagnostic techniques hold great promise for patients with epilepsy.

One of the early reports on the use of computer-assisted tomography (CT) stated that the machine 'adds a new dimension to patient care and may well revolutionize the practice of neuroradiology' (Baker et al., 1974). Indeed, the use of CT has altered the way neurologists, neurosurgeons, and neuroradiologists diagnose changes in the density of abnormal brain structures. Although epileptic patients with demonstrable density-altering lesions have benefited greatly from these studies, many other patients have subtle changes in physiologic function without changes in brain density at the site of the lesion. In these patients, the CT scan serves only to rule out a lesion such as a tumor. Patients may have severe epilepsy but not have CT scan abnormalities. In 23 patients with intractable seizures, for example, only three had CT scan abnormalities, even with contrast enhancement (Porter et al., 1977).

The technique of positron emission tomography (PET) appears to be especially suited for the study and evaluation of partial epilepsy. Whereas the CT scan is a measure of brain density, with changes most apparent at tissue-fluid or tissue-bone interfaces, the PET scan is a measure of regional changes in physiologic function, specifically metabolism and blood flow. The CT scan uses exogenous X-ray penetration of the brain, like a conventional roentgenogram. The PET scan uses radioactive emission of an intravenously injected nuclide, much like a brain scan. The differential distribution of the nuclide in the brain is a function of metabolic activity or blood flow or other physiologic factors. The advantage of the PET scan over the brain scan is its ability to localize by 'slices,' as in a CT scan. The disadvantage is the expense of the apparatus and the remarkably short half-life of the isotopes utilized in the technique.

Considerable data on the PET technique strongly suggest its important role in the diagnosis and treatment of epilepsy, especially of patients with severe partial seizures. The following conclusions (Engel et al., 1982a, 1982b,

1982c; Newmark et al., 1982; Theodore et al., 1983c) appear to be reasonable at this stage of development of the technique:

1. Localized epileptic lesions usually show altered glucose metabolism at the site of the epileptogenic focus (with fluorodeoxyglucose as the nuclide). Metabolism at the abnormal site is usually decreased (hypometabolic) between seizures and increased (hypermetabolic) during seizures.

2. Patients with generalized seizures, such as absence attacks, usually do not have localized metabolic changes demonstrated by PET.

3. Aside from localization, EEG abnormalities, such as spikes, do not correlate quantitatively with the PET scan, suggesting that the two techniques measure different aspects of cerebral dysfunction.

4. In general, the PET technique is useful in the evaluation of patients with severe partial seizures who are surgical candidates. Only personnel and equipment costs (one must, for example, have access to a cyclotron) prohibit its widespread use in such patients.

Another new technique with strong potential benefit in epilepsy is nuclear magnetic resonance (NMR). Whereas CT scanners are sensitive only to the elemental composition of tissue, NMR scanners are primarily sensitive to the chemical environment of hydrogen in the tissue. Greater differentiation is possible, for example, between white and gray matter (Doyle et al., 1981). The possibilities for better and better resolution of scans and, eventually, physiologic studies as well, make the NMR technique a promising advance in brain imaging.

Finally, a completely different diagnostic tool, the magnetoencephalogram (MEG), might eventually be one of the most powerful of all measuring devices of the physiologic function of the brain. Ever since the beginning of electroencephalography, interpreters of EEGs have interpreted the scalp recordings as reflecting primarily cortical activity and only indirectly activity from deeper structures. Attempts to get closer to critical structures resulted in sphenoidal and nasopharyngeal recording, and ultimately, in relatively few patients, depth electrode placement by surgical procedures to record deeper structures. Clearly what is needed is a noninvasive method for obtaining information on the bioelectric activity of the brain at all levels, not just at the surface. Although electrical fields generated in the depths of the brain are not transmitted adequately to surface electrodes, the associated magnetic fields, though weak, are transmitted undiminished through brain, skull and scalp. The development of an extremely sensitive magnetometer, the 'super-conducting quantum interference device' (referred to as the SQUID), makes possible the measurement of magnetic fields of the brain. The MEG technique has been used to record the location, depth, orientation, and polarity of magnetic spike field strength in epileptic patients (Barth et al., 1982). Improvements in the number of channels, instrument sensitivity, and data display seem likely, as do the possible benefits to patients with epilepsy.

Appendix

Chapters of the International League Against Epilepsy
and the International Bureau for Epilepsy

The International League Against Epilepsy (ILAE) is primarily a professional organization, and the International Bureau for Epilepsy (IBE) is an organization with both lay and professional members. The purpose of this appendix is to guide physicians to expertise in epilepsy in their various countries, through the ILAE and IBE national chapters. This list, provided by Epilepsy International (EI), a joint effort of ILAE and IBE, is accurate as of early 1983. Permission to print this list has been granted by Epilepsy International. Publication of the list does not in any way imply endorsement of this volume by ILAE or IBE or their various chapters or by EI.

ARGENTINA

(ILAE)
Liga Argentina contra la Epilepsia
Gelly y Obes 2247
1425 Buenos Aires

(IBE)
Associacion de Lucha contra la Epilepsia
Tucuman 3261
Buenos Aires 1189

AUSTRALIA

(IBE)
National Committee on Epilepsy
P.O. Box 554
Lilydale, Vic. 3140

AUSTRIA

(ILAE)
The Chapter of ILAE in Austria
Lazarettgasse, 14
A-1090 Vienna

BELGIUM

(IBE)
Les Amis de la Ligue National Belge contre l'Epilepsie
135 Avenue Albert
Brussels 1060

BOLIVIA

(ILAE)
The Chapter of ILAE in Bolivia
Casilla 3370
La Paz

BRAZIL

(ILAE)
Liga Brasileira de Epilepsia
SQS 307 B. D Ap. 303-70354
Brasilia, D.F.

CANADA

(ILAE)
Canadian League Against Epilepsy
The University of British Columbia
2075 Wesbrook Mall
Vancouver, BC V6T 1W5

(IBE)
Epilepsy Canada
2145 Lakeshore Dr.
Dorval, Quebec H9S 2G4

CHILE

(ILAE)
Liga Chilena contra la Epilepsia
Los Ceibos 2236
Santiago

(IBE)
Liga Contra la Epilepsia de Valparaiso
PO Box 150, Vina del Mar

COLOMBIA

(ILAE)
Liga Central contra la Epilepsia
Apartado Aereo 057751
Bogota, D.E.

(IBE)
Liga Colombiana contra la Epilepsia
Apdo. Aereo 604
Cartagena

CZECHOSLOVAKIA

(ILAE)
Czechoslovak League Against Epilepsy
Marothyho, 1
811 06 Bratislava

DENMARK

(ILAE)
Danish Epilepsy Society
Rorholmsgade 22, 5/th
DK—1352 Copenhagen K

(IBE)
Epilepsikliniken, Odense Sygehus
5000 Odense C
   (and)
Dansk Epilepsiforening
Admiralgade 15
1066 Copenhagen K

DOMINICAN REPUBLIC

(ILAE)
Sociedad Dominicana contra la Epilepsia
The Amado Garcia Querrero No. 233
Santo Domingo

EAST GERMANY

(ILAE)
The Chapter of ILAE in East Germany
Vors, der Gesselschaft fur Neuroelektro-diagnostik der DDR
Direktor der Nervenklinik der Ernst-Moritz-Arndt-Universitat
DDR—22 Greifswald

FINLAND

(ILAE)
Finnish Epilepsy Association
Dept. of Neurology
University of Kuopio
70210 Kuopio

(IBE)
Epilepsialiitto r.y.
Lapinrinne 2
00180 Helsinki 18
  (and)
KYKY neur. Pkl.
70210 Kuopio 21

FRANCE

(ILAE)
Ligue Francaise contre l'Epilepsie
Etablissement Medical de la Teppe
26600 Tain-L'Hermitage
  (and)
Clinique Neurologique
Hopital Saint Julian
1, Rue Foller
54037 Nancy Cedex

(IBE)
Groupe de Recherches et d'informations du nord sur l'Epilepsie
11, Avenue du President Kennedy
59800 Lille

WEST GERMANY

(ILAE)
German League Against Epilepsy
Klinikum Charlottenburg
Freie Universitat Berlin
Spandauer Damm 130
D-1000 Berlin 19

(and)
Neurologishe Klinik
Fakultat fur Klinische Medizin Mannheim
Universitat Heidelberg
Theodor-Kutzer-Ufer
6800 Mannheim, 1

(IBE)
Interessenvereinigung fur Ansfallskranke e.v.
Hochfeld 21b
8134 Pocking
   (and)
Stiftung Michael
Karthauserstrasse, 10
5300 Bonn, 1

GREAT BRITAIN

(ILAE)
The Chapter of ILAE in Great Britain
27 Clarendon Rd.
Leeds LS2 9NZ, West Yorkshire
   (and)
Univ. Dept. of Neurology
King's College Hospital
Denmark Hill, London SE5 9RS

(IBE)
British Epilepsy Association
North Regional Centre
313 Chapeltown Road
Leeds LS7 3LT

GREECE

(IBE)
Greek National Association Against Epilepsy
45 Solonos St.
Athens 134

INDIA

(IBE)
The Indian Epilepsy Association
251, D. Dadobhoy Naoroji Rd.
Fort Bombay 400 001

IRELAND

(IBE)
Irish Epilepsy Association
249 Crumlin Rd.
Dublin 12

ISRAEL

(ILAE)
The Israel League Against Epilepsy
PO Box 9611
Haifa

ITALY

(ILAE)
Lega Italiana contro l'Epilessia
Via U. Foscolo, 7
40123 Bologna
   (and)
Istituto Neurologica 'Besta'
Via Celoria 11
20133 Milano

(IBE)
Federazione Italiana delle Associazioni Regionali per la lotta
   contro l'Epilessia
Via Plinio, 40
20129 Milano
   (and)
Via Einaudi 23
57037 Portoferrario (Livorno)
Isola d'Elba

JAPAN

(ILAE)
The Japanese Epilepsy Society
National Musashi Research Institute for Mental and Nervous
   Disease
2620 Ogawa-Higashi
Kodaira (MZ 187) Tokyo

(IBE)
The Japanese Epilepsy Association
5F Zenkokuzaidan Bldg.
2-2-8 Nishiwaseda, Shinjuku-ku
Tokyo, 162

KOREA

(IBE)
Korean Epilepsy Association
204-1 Yeonhi-Dong
Seodaemun-Kun
Seoul 120

MEXICO
(ILAE)
Mexican League Against Epilepsy
Insurgentes Sur No. 3877
Col. La Fama, Deleg. Tlalpan
14410 Mexico, D.F.

THE NETHERLANDS

(ILAE)
The Chapter of ILAE in Netherlands
Instituut voor Epilepsiebestrijding
Achterweg 5, 2103 SW Heemstede
    (and)
Epilepsiecentrum 'Kempenhaeghe'
Sterkselseweg 65
5591 VE Heeze

(IBE)
Epilepsie Vereniging Nederland
Konigslaan 19
3583 GD Utrecht

NEW ZEALAND

(IBE)
New Zealand Epilepsy Association
PO Box 190
Dunedin

NORWAY

(ILAE)
The Chapter of ILAE in Norway
Statens Center for Epilepsi
PO Box 900
1301 Sandvika

(and)
Director, Statens Center for Epilepsy
N-1301 Sandvika

(IBE)
Norsk Epilepsiforbund
Kristian August gt, 19,
Oslo 1
  (and)
National Epilepsy Center
Solbergv. 23
N-1301 Sandvika

POLAND

(ILAE)
The Chapter of ILAE in Poland
Dept. of Neurology
Research and Training Center of Medical Academy
ul Grenadierow 51/59
04-073 Warsaw

PORTUGAL

(ILAE)
The Chapter of ILAE in Portugal
R. Con. de Sabugosa 29-3E
Lisbon, 5

(IBE)
Liga Nacional Portuguesa contra la Epilepsia
Rue Joao, Penha, 14-B
1200 Lisbon

SOUTH AFRICA

(IBE)
South African National Epilepsy League
PO Box 200
Springs 1560
  (and)
Jan Kriel Institute and School
PO Box 17,
Kuilsrivier 7580, Cape Province

SPAIN

(ILAE)
Liga Espanola contra la Epilepsia
Platon 3,3,1
Barcelona 2
  (and)
c/o Manila, 57,60,2a
Barcelona, 34

(IBE)
Patronata contra las Enfermedades Neurologicas Paroxisticas
Felipe II 192
Barcelona

SWEDEN

(ILAE)
The Chapter of ILAE in Sweden
13 Bagargrand
S-123 54 Farsta

SWITZERLAND

(ILAE)
The Chapter of ILAE in Switzerland
Pro Infirmis, Postfach 129
8032 Zurich
  (and)
Med. Universitats-Kinderklinik und Poliklinik
Inselspital Bern
Freiburgstrasse 23
3010 Bern

TURKEY

(IBE)
Turkish Epilepsy Association
Necatibey Caddesi No. 19-6
Yenesehire, Ankara

UNITED STATES OF AMERICA

(ILAE)
The American Epilepsy Society
179 Allyn St., Suite 304
Hartford, CT 06103

(IBE)
Epilepsy Foundation of America
4351 Garden City Drive
Landover, MD 20785

URUGUAY

(ILAE)
Liga Uruguaya contra la Epilepsia
Instituto de Neurologia, P. 2
Hospital de Clinicas
Montevideo

Bibliography

Adams, R.D., & Foley, J.M. (1953) The neurological disorder associated with liver disease. *Proceedings of the Association for Research in Nervous and Mental Disease*, 32, 198-237.

Aicardi, J. & Chevrie, J.J. (1983) Consequences of status epilepticus in infants and children. In *Advances in Neurology, Vol 34: Status Epilepticus—Mechanisms of Brain Damage and Treatment* (Ed.) Delgado-Escueta, A.V., Wasterlain, C.G., Treiman, D.M. & Porter, R.J. pp.115-125. New York: Raven Press.

American Psychiatric Association (1980) *Diagnostic and Statistical Manual of Mental Disorders*, Third Edition. Washington, D.C.: APA. pp.253-260.

Aminoff, M.J., & Simon, R.P. (1980) Status epilepticus: Causes, clinical features, and consequences in 98 patients. *American Journal of Medicine*, 69, 657-666.

Andermann, F. & Robb, J.P. (1972) Absence status: A reappraisal following review of thirty-eight patients. *Epilepsia*, 13, 177-187.

Asconape, J. & Penry, J.K. (1983) Some clinical and EEG aspects of benign juvenile myoclonic epilepsy. *Epilepsia*, 24, 246.

Ayala, G.F., Matsumoto, H. & Gumnit, R.J. (1970) Excitability changes and inhibitory mechanisms in neocortical neurons during seizures. *Journal of Neurophysiology*, 33, 73-85.

Baker H.L., Campbell, J.K., Houser, O.W., Reese, D.F., Sheedy, P.F., Holman, C.B. & Kurland, R.L. (1974) Computer assisted tomography of the head: An early evaluation. *Mayo Clinic Proceedings*, 49, 17-27.

Barth, D.S., Sutherling, W., Engel, J., Jr. & Beatty, J. (1982) Neuromagnetic localization of epileptiform spike activity in the human brain. *Science*, 218, 891-894.

Baruzzi, A. Michelucci, R. & Tassinari, C.A. (1982) Benzodiazepines: Nitrazepam. In *Antiepileptic Drugs*, Second Edition (Ed.) Woodbury, D.M., Penry, J.K. & Pippenger, C.E. pp.753-769. New York: Raven Press.

Bazemore, R.P. & Zuckermann, E.C. (1974) On the problem of diphenylhydantoin-induced seizures: An experimental approach. *Archives of Neurology*, 31, 243-249.

Beaussart M. & Faou, R. (1978) Evolution of epilepsy with rolandic paroxysmal foci: A study of 324 cases. *Epilepsia*, 19, 337-342.

Bjerkedal, T., Czeizel, A., Goujard, J., Kallen, B., Mastroiacova, P., Nevin, N., Oakley, G. & Robert, E. (1982) Valproic acid and spina bifida. *Lancet*, 2, 1096.

Booker, H.E. (1982a) Trimethadione: Relation of plasma concentration to seizure control. In *Antiepileptic Drugs*, Second Edition (Ed.) Woodbury, D.M., Penry, J.K. & Pippenger, C.E. pp.697-699. New York: Raven Press.

Booker, H.E. (1982b) Trimethadione: Toxicity. In *Antiepileptic Drugs*, Second Edition (Ed.) Woodbury, D.M., Penry, J.K. & Pippenger, C.E. pp.701-703. New York: Raven Press.

Boshes, L.D. & Gibbs, F.A. (1972) *Epilepsy Handbook*, Second Edition. Springfield, Ill.: Charles C Thomas. 196 pp.

Bourgeois, F.D.B., Dodson, W.E. & Ferrendelli, J.A. (1982) Primidone (PRM), phenobarbital (PB), and PEMA: Seizure protection, neurotoxicity, and therapeutic index (TI) of each single compound. *Neurology*, 32, A224.

Browne, T.R., (1978) Drug therapy reviews: Drug therapy of status epilepticus. *American Journal of Hospital Pharmacy*, 35, 915-922.

Browne, T.R., Penry, J.K., Porter, R.J. & Dreifuss, F.E. (1974) Responsiveness before, during, and after spike-wave paroxysms. *Neurology*, 24, 659-665.

Browne, T.R., Dreifuss, F.E., Dyken, P.R., Goode, D.J., Penry, J.K., Porter R.J., White, B.G. & White P.T. (1975) Ethosuximide in the treatment of absence (petit mal) seizures. *Neurology*, 25, 515-524.

Camerman, A. & Camerman, N. (1980) Structure-activity relationships: Stereochemical similarities in chemically different antiepileptic drugs. In *Antiepileptic Drugs: Mechanisms of Action* (Ed.) Glaser, G.H., Penry, J.K. & Woodbury, D.M. pp.223-231. New York: Raven Press.

Cereghino, J.J. & Penry, J.K. (1982) General principles. Testing of antiepileptic drugs in humans: Clinical considerations. In *Antiepileptic Drugs*, Second Edition (Ed.) Woodbury, D.M., Penry, J.K. & Pippenger, C.E. pp.141-157. New York: Raven Press.

Cereghino, J.J., Penry, J.K. & Smith, L.D. (1980) Comprehensive epilepsy programs in the United States. In *Advances in Epileptology: XIth Epilepsy International Symposium* (Ed.) Canger, R., Angeleri, F. & Penry, J.K. pp.257-260. New York: Raven Press.

Cereghino, J.J., Brock, J.T., Van Meter, J.C., Penry, J.K., Smith, L.D. & White, B.G. (1974) Carbamazepine for epilepsy: A controlled prospective evaluation. *Neurology*, 24, 401-410.

Charleton, M.H., editor (1975) *Myoclonic Seizures*. Amsterdam: Exerpta Medica. 167 pp.

Christiansen, C., Brandt, N.J., Ebbesen, F., Sardemann, H. & Trolle, D. (1980) Do newborns of epileptics on anticonvulsants develop biochemical signs of osteomalacia? A controlled prospective study. *Acta Neurologica Scandinavica*, 62, 158-164.

Ciesielski, L., Maitre, M., Cash, C. & Mandel, P. (1975) Regional distribution in brain and effect on cerebral mitochondrial respiration of the anticonvulsive drug n-Dipropylacetate. *Biochemical Pharmacology*, 24, 1055-1058.

Cloyd, J.C., Gumnit, R.J. & McLain, L.W., Jr. (1980) Status epilepticus: The role of intravenous phenytoin. *Journal of the American Medical Association*, 244, 1479-1481.

Commission for the Control of Epilepsy and Its Consequences (1978) *Plan for Nationwide Action on Epilepsy*, Vol 1. DHEW Publication No. (NIH) 78-276. Washington, D.C.: U.S. Department of Health Education and Welfare.

Commission on Classification and Terminology of the International League Against Epilepsy (1981) Proposal for revised clinical and electroencephalographic classification of epileptic seizures. *Epilepsia*, 22, 489-501.

Cramer, J.A. & Mattson, R.H. (1979) Valproic acid: *In vitro* plasma protein binding and interaction with phenytoin. *Therapeutic Drug Monitoring*, 1, 105-116.

Daly, D.D. (1975) Ictal clinical manifestations of complex partial seizures. In *Advances in Neurology, Vol 11: Complex Partial Seizures and Their Treatment* (Ed.) Penry, J.K. & Daly, D.D. pp.57-83. New York: Raven Press.

Dam, M. (1982) Phenytoin: Toxicity. In *Antiepileptic Drugs*, Second Edition (Ed.) Woodbury, D.M., Penry, J.K. & Pippenger, C.E. pp.247-256. New York: Raven Press.

De Jong, R.N. (1977) Case taking and the neurologic examination. In *Clinical Neurology* (Ed.) Baker, A.B. & Baker, L.H. pp.1-83. Hagerstown: Harper & Row.

Delgado-Escueta, A., Ferrendelli, J. & Prince, D. (1983) Cellular communication in epilepsy. *Annals of Neurology* [Suppl] (in press).

Delgado-Escueta, A.V., Bacsal, F.E. & Treiman, D.M. (1981a) Complex partial seizures on closed-circuit television and EEG: A study of 691 attacks in 79 patients. *Annals of Neurology*, 11, 292-300.

Delgado-Escueta, A.V., Mattson, R.H., King, L., Goldensohn, E.S., Spiegel, H., Madsen, J., Crandall, P., Dreifuss, F. & Porter, R.J. (1981b) The nature of aggression during epileptic seizures. *New England Journal of Medicine*, 305, 711-716.

Delgado-Escueta, A.V., Wasterlain, C., Treiman, D.M. & Porter, R.J. (1982) Current concepts in neurology: Management of status epilepticus. *New England Journal of Medicine*, 306, 1337-1340.

Desai, B.T., Porter, R.J. & Penry, J.K. (1982) Psychogenic seizures: A study of 42 attacks in six patients, with intensive monitoring. *Archives of Neurology*, 39, 202-209.

Desai, B.T., Riley, T.L., Porter, R.J. & Penry, J.K. (1978) Active noncompliance as a cause of uncontrolled seizures. *Epilepsia*, 19, 447-452.

Doyle, F.H., Pennock, J.M., Orr, J.S., Gore, J.C., Bydder, G.M., Steiner, R.E., Young, I.R., Clow, H., Bailes, D.R., Burl, M., Gilderdale, D.J. & Walters, P.E. (1981) Imaging of the brain by nuclear magnetic resonance. *Lancet*, 2, 53-57.

Dreifuss, F.E. (1982) Ethosuximide: Toxicity. In *Antiepileptic Drugs*, Second Edition (Ed.) Woodbury, D.M., Penry, J.K. & Pippenger, C.E. pp.647-653. New York: Raven Press.

Dreifuss, F.E. & Sato, S. (1982) Benzodiazepines: Clonazepam. In *Antiepileptic Drugs*, Second Edition (Ed.) Woodbury, D.M., Penry, J.K. & Pippenger, C.E. pp.737-752. New York: Raven Press.

Easton, J.D. & Sherman, D.G. (1976) Somatic anxiety attacks and propranolol. *Archives of Neurology*, 33, 689-691.

Efron, R. (1961) Post-epileptic paralysis: Theoretical critique and report of a case. *Brain*, 84, 381-394.

Ehrenberg, B.L. & Penry, J.K. (1976) Computer recognition of generalized spike-wave discharges. *Electroencephalography and Clinical Neurophysiology*, 41, 25-36.

Eilers, R.D. & Melone, J.J. (undated) The underwriting and rating of workmen's compensation insurance—with particular reference to the coverage of employees afflicted with epilepsy. Washington, D.C.: The Epilepsy Foundation. 16 pp.

Emerson, R., D'Souza, B.J., Vining, E.P., Holden, K.R., Mellits, E.D. & Freeman, J.M. (1981) Stopping medication in children with epilepsy: Predictors of outcome. *New England Journal of Medicine*, 304, 1125-1129.

Engel, J.,Jr., Ludwig, B.I. & Fetell, M. (1978) Prolonged partial complex status epilepticus: EEG and behavioral observations. *Neurology*, 28, 863-869.

Engel, J.,Jr., Kuhl, D.E., Phelps, M.E. & Crandall, P.H. (1982a) Comparative localization of epileptic foci in partial epilepsy by PCT and EEG. *Annals of Neurology*, 12, 529-537.

Engel, J.,Jr., Kuhl D.E., Phelps, M.E. & Mazziotta, J.C. (1982b) Interictal cerebral glucose metabolism in partial epilepsy and its relation to EEG changes. *Annals of Neurology* 12, 510-517.

Engel, J.,Jr., Brown, W.J., Kuhl, D.E., Phelps, M.E., Mazziotta, J.C. & Crandall, P.H. (1982c) Pathological findings underlying focal hypometabolism in partial epilepsy. *Annals of Neurology*, 12, 518-528.

Escueta, A.V., Kunze, U., Waddell, G, Boxley, J. & Nadel, A. (1977) Lapse of consciousness and automatisms in temporal lobe epilepsy: A videotape analysis. *Neurology*, 27, 144-155.

Fenichel, G.M. (1980) *Neonatal Neurology*. New York: Churchill Livingstone. pp.20-44.

Fishman, R.A. (1980) *Cerebrospinal Fluid in Diseases of the Nervous System*. Philadelphia: W.B. Saunders. 384 pp.

Food and Drug Administration (1981) New standards for phenytoin products. *FDA Drug Bulletin*, 11, 4.

Forster, F.M. & Booker, H.E. (1975) The epilepsies and convulsive disorders. In *Clinical Neurology, Vol 2* (Ed.) Baker, A.B. & Baker, L.H. Chapter 24. Hagerstown: Harper and Row.

Frost, J.D., Hrachovy, R.A., Kellaway. P. & Zion T. (1978) Quantitative analysis and characterization of infantile spasms. *Epilepsia*, 19, 273-282.

Gastaut, H. (1968) Semeiologie des myoclonies et nosologie analytique des syndromes myocloniques. In *Les Myoclonies* (Ed.) Bonduelle, M. & Gastaut, H. pp.1-30. Paris: Masson.

Gastaut, H. (1970) Clinical and electroencephalographic classification of epileptic seizures. *Epilepsia*, 11, 102-113.

Gastaut, H. (1973) *Dictionary of Epilepsy*. Geneva: World Health Organization. 75 pp.

Gastaut, H. (1983) Classification of status epilepticus. In *Advances in Neurology, Vol. 34: Status Epilepticus—Mechanisms of Brain Damage and Treatment* (Ed.) Delgado-Escueta, A.V., Wasterlain, C.G., Treiman, D.M. & Porter, R.J. pp.15-35. New York: Raven Press.

Gastaut, H. & Villeneuve, A. (1967) The startle disease or hyperekplexia: Pathological surprise reaction. *Journal of the Neurological Sciences*, 5, 523-542.

Gastaut, H. & Broughton, R. (1972) *Epileptic Seizures: Clinical and Electrographic Features, Diagnosis and Treatment*. Springfield, Ill.: Charles C Thomas. 286 pp.

Gastaut, H., Roger, J., Soulayrol, R., Tassinari, C.A., Regis, H., Dravet, C., Bernard, R., Pinsard, N. & Saint-Jean, M. (1966) Childhood epileptic encephalopathy with diffuse slow spike-waves (otherwise known as 'petit mal variant') or Lennox syndrome. *Epilepsia*, 7, 139-179.

Gloor, P., Olivier, A. & Ives, J. (1980) Loss of consciousness in temporal lobe seizures: Observations obtained with stereotaxic depth electrode recordings and stimulations. In *Advances in Epileptology: XIth Epilepsy International Symposium* (Ed.) Canger, R., Angeleri, F. & Penry, J.K. pp. 349-353. New York: Raven Press.

Goldberg, M.A. (1982) Eterobarb: Absorption, distribution, biotransformation, and excretion. In *Antiepileptic Drugs*, Second Edition (Ed.) Woodbury, D.M., Penry, J.K. & Pippenger, C.E. pp. 803-811. New York: Raven Press.

Goldstein, D.S., Spanarkel, M., Pitterman, A., Toltzis, R., Gratz, E., Epstein, S. & Keiser, H.R. (1982) Circulatory control mechanisms in vasodepressor syncope. *American Heart Journal*, 104, 1071-1075.

Gowers, W.R. (1885) *Epilepsy and Other Chronic Convulsive Diseases: Their Causes, Symptoms & Treatment*. Reprint. New York: Dover Publications, 1964. 255 pp.

Gratz, E.S., Theodore, W.H., Newmark, M.E., Kupferberg, H.J., Porter, R.J. & Qu, Z. (1982) Effect of carbamazepine on phenytoin clearance in patients with complex partial seizures. *Neurology*, 32, A223.

Gumnit, R.J., editor, and Sell, M.A., associate editor (1981) *Epilepsy: A Handbook for Physicians*, Fourth Edition. Minneapolis: University of Minnesota Comprehensive Epilepsy Program. 64 pp.

Halliday, A.M. (1967) The clinical incidence of myoclonus. In *Modern Trends in Neurology, Vol 4* (Ed.) Williams, D. pp.69-105. London: Butterworths.

Hanson J.W. & Smith, D.W. (1975) The fetal hydantoin syndrome. *Journal of Pediatrics*, 87, 285-290.

Hanson, J.W. & Buehler, B.A. (1982) Fetal hydantoin syndrome: Current status. *Journal of Pediatrics*, 101, 816-818.

Harper, M. & Roth, M. (1962) Temporal lobe epilepsy and the phobic anxiety-depersonalization syndrome. Part I: A comparative study. *Comprehensive Psychiatry*, 3, 129-151.

Hauser, W.A. (1981) The natural history of febrile seizures. In *Febrile Seizures* (Ed.) Nelson, K.B. & Ellenberg, J.H. pp.5-17. New York: Raven Press.

Hauser, W.A., Annegers, J.F. & Elveback, L.R. (1980) Mortality in patients with epilepsy. *Epilepsia*, 21, 399-412.

Homan, R.W. & Walker, J.E. (1983) Clinical studies of lorazepam in status epilepticus. In *Advances in Neurology, Vol 34: Status Epilepticus—Mechanisms of Brain Damage and Treatment* (Ed.) Delgado-Escueta, A.V., Wasterlain, C.G., Treiman, D.M. & Porter, R.J. pp.493-498. New York: Raven Press.

Hrachovy, R.A. (1982) Infantile spasms. In *Classification of the Epilepsies: Age Related Syndromic Seizure Types. State of the Science in EEG and Epilepsy.* Annual Meeting of the American EEG Society and the American Epilepsy Society, Phoenix, 1982.

Ives, J.R., Thompson, C.J. & Gloor, P. (1976) Seizure monitoring: A new tool in electro-encephalography. *Electroencephalography and Clinical Neurophysiology*, 41, 422-427.

Jackson, J.H., (1888) On a particular variety of epilepsy ('intellectual aura'), one case with symptoms of organic brain disease. *Brain*, 11, 179-207.

Janz, D. (1983) Etiology of convulsive status epilepticus. In *Advances in Neurology, Vol 34: Status Epilepticus—Mechanisms of Brain Damage and Treatment* (Ed.) Delgado-Escueta, A.V., Wasterlain, C.G., Treiman, D.M. & Porter, R.J. pp.47-54. New York: Raven Press.

Janz, D. & Christian, W., (1957) Impulsiv-Petit mal. *Deutsche Zeitschrift fur Nervenheilkunde*, 176, 346-386.

Janz, D. & Beck-Mannagetta, G. (1981) Abnormalities of delivery, gestation, and postnatal period in the offspring of epileptic parents: Retrospective study. *Epilepsia*, 22, 373.

Jeavons, P.M. (1977) Nosological problems of myoclonic epilepsies in childhood and adolescence. *Developmental Medicine and Child Neurology*, 19, 3-8.

Jeavons, P.M., Clark, J.E. & Maheshwari, M.C. (1977) Treatment of generalized epilepsies of childhood and adolescence with sodium valproate ('Epilim'). *Developmental Medicine and Child Neurology*, 19, 9-25.

Jones, T.D. & Jacobs, J.L. (1932) The treatment of obstinate chorea with Nirvanol. *Journal of the American Medical Association*, 99, 18-21.

Jusko, W.J., (1976) Bioavailability and disposition kinetics of phenytoin in man. In *Quantitative Analytic Studies In Epilepsy* (Ed.) Kellaway, P. & Petersen, I. pp.115-136. New York: Raven Press.

Kaneko, S., Suzuki, K., Sato, T., Ogawa, Y. & Nowura, Y. (1981) The problems of antiepileptic medication in the neonatal period: Is breast feeding advisable? *Epilepsia*, 22, 375.

Kapetanovic, I., Kupferberg, H.J., Porter, R.J. & Penry, J.K. (1980) Valproic acid—phenobarbital interaction: A systematic study using stable isotopically labelled phenobarbital in an epileptic patient. In *Antiepileptic Therapy: Advances in Drug Monitoring* (Ed.) Johannessen, S.I., Morselli, P.L., Pippenger, C.E., Richens, A., Schmidt, D. & Meinardi, H. pp.373-380. New York: Raven Press.

Kapetanovic, I.M., Kupferberg, H.J., Porter, R.J., Theodore, W., Schulman, E. & Penry, J.K. (1981) Mechanism of valproate-phenobarbital interaction in epileptic patients. *Clinical Pharmacology and Therapeutics*, 29, 480-486.

Kellaway, P., Hrachovy, R.A., Frost, J.D. & Zion, T. (1979) A precise characterization and quantification of infantile spasms. *Annals of Neurology*, 6, 214-218.

Kelly, E.C. (1939) John Hughlings Jackson. *Medical Classics*, 3, 915.

Kendig, E.L.,Jr., Dyken, P.R., Hernandez, N., McKee, M.C., Peterson, H., Richards, N.G., Shackelford, R.H., Smith, E.E., Wilder, B.J. & Wittes, J. (1981) Consensus statement on febrile seizures. In *Febrile Seizures* (Ed.) Nelson, K.B. & Ellenberg, J.H. pp.301-306. New York: Raven Press.

Kiloh, L.G., McComas, A.J., Osselton, J.W. & Upton, A.R.M. (1981) *Clinical Electroencephalography*, Fourth Edition. London: Butterworths. 292 pp.

Klass, D.W. & Daly, D.D. (1979) *Current Practice of Clinical Electroencephalography*. New York: Raven Press. 532 pp.

Klawans, H.L. (1979) *Clinical Neuropharmacology, Vol 4*. New York: Raven Press. 228 pp.

Kooi, K.A., Tucker, R.P. & Marshall, R.E. (1978) *Fundamentals of Electroencephalography*, Second Edition. Hagerstown: Harper & Row. 249 pp.

Krall, R.L., Penry, J.K., Kupferberg, H.J. & Swinyard, E.A. (1978a) Antiepileptic drug development: I. History and a program for progress. *Epilepsia*, 19, 393-408.

Krall, R.L., Penry, J.K., White, B.G., Kupferberg, H.J. & Swinyard, E.A. (1978b) Antiepileptic drug development: II. Anticonvulsant drug screening. *Epilepsia*, 19, 409-428.

Kupferberg, H.J. (1980) Sodium valproate. In *Advances in Neurology, Vol 27: Antiepileptic Drugs—Mechanisms of Action* (Ed.) Glaser, G.H., Penry, J.K. & Woodbury, D.M. pp.643-654. New York: Raven Press.

Kupferberg, H.J. (1982) Other hydantoins: Mephenytoin and ethotoin. In *Antiepileptic Drugs*, Second Edition (Ed.) Woodbury, D.M., Penry, J.K & Pippenger, C.E. pp.283-295. New York: Raven Press.

Kupferberg, H.J. & Penry, J.K. (1975) The development of a matrix reference standard for anti-epileptic analysis. In *Clinical Pharmacology of Anti-epileptic Drugs* (Ed.) Schneider, H., Janz, D., Gardner-Thorpe, C., Meinardi, H. & Sherwin, A.L. pp.304-306. Berlin: Springer-Verlag.

Kupferberg, H.J. & Yonekawa, W. (1975) The metabolism of 3-methyl-5-ethyl-5-phenylhydantoin (mephenytoin) to 5-ethyl-5-phenylhydantoin (Nirvanol) in mice in relation to anticonvulsant activity. *Drug Metabolism and Disposition*, 3, 26-29.

Kupferberg, H.J. & Longacre-Shaw, J. (1979) Mephobarbital and phenobarbital plasma concentrations in epileptic patients treated with mephobarbital. *Therapeutic Drug Monitoring*, 1, 117-122.

Kupferberg, H.J., Yonekawa, W.D., Newmark, M.E., Porter, R.J. & Penry, J.K. (1978) Measurement of mephenytoin and its demethylated metabolite, Nirvanol, by mass fragmentography in epileptic patients. *Abstracts of the 7th International Congress of Pharmacology*. Paris, 1978. p.181.

Kutt, H. (1982) Phenytoin: Relation of plasma concentration to seizure control. In *Antiepileptic Drugs*, Second Edition (Ed.) Woodbury, D.M., Penry, J.K. & Pippenger, C.E. pp. 241-246. New York: Raven Press.

Kutt, H., Winters, W., Kokenge, R. & McDowell, F. (1964) Diphenylhydantoin metabolism, blood levels, and toxicity. *Archives of Neurology*, 11, 642-648.

Lacy, J.R. & Penry, J.K. (1976) *Infantile Spasms*. New York: Raven Press. 169 pp.

Lai, C. & Ziegler, D.K. (1981) Syncope problem solved by continuous ambulatory simultaneous EEG/ECG recording. *Neurology*, 31, 1152-1154.

Lance, J.W. & Adams, R.D. (1963) The syndrome of intention or action myoclonus as a sequel to hypoxic encephalophathy. *Brain*, 86, 111-140.

Lennox, W.G. (1945) The petit mal epilepsies: Their treatment with Tridione. *Journal of the American Medical Association*, 129, 1069-1074.

Lennox, W.G. (1960) *Epilepsy and Related Disorders, Vol 1*. Boston: Little, Brown. 574 pp.

Lerman, P. & Kivity, S. (1982) The efficacy of corticotropin in primary infantile spasms. *Journal of Pediatrics*, 101, 294-296.

Lombroso, C.T. (1967) Sylvian seizures and midtemporal spike foci in children. *Archives of Neurology*, 17, 52-59.

Louis, S., Kutt, H. & McDowell, F. (1967) The cardiocirculatory changes caused by intravenous Dilantin and its solvent. *American Heart Journal*, 74, 523-529.

Marsden, C.D. (1976) Neurology. In *A Textbook of Epilepsy* (Ed.) Laidlaw, J. & Richens, A. pp.15-65. Edinburgh: Churchill Livingstone.

Marsden, C.D., Hallet, M. & Fahn, S. (1982) The nosology and pathophysiology of myoclonus. In *Neurology 2: Movement Disorders* (Ed.) Marsden, C.D. & Fahn, S. pp.196-248. London: Butterworths.

Masland, R.L. (1975) A controlled trial of clonazepam in temporal lobe epilepsy. *Acta Neurologica Scandinavica (Suppl.)*, 75, 49-54.

Matthews, W.B. (1976) Paroxysmal symptoms in multiple sclerosis. *Journal of Neurology, Neurosurgery, and Psychiatry*, 38, 617-623.

Mattson, R.H. (1980) Value of intensive monitoring. In *Advances in Epileptology: The Xth Epilepsy International Symposium* (Ed.) Wada, J.A. & Penry, J.K. pp.43-51. New York: Raven Press.

Mattson, R.H., Klein, P.E., Caldwell, B.V. & Cramer, J.A. (1982) Medroxy progesterone treatment of women with uncontrolled seizures. *Epilepsia*, 23, 436-437.

Maynert, E.W. (1972) Phenobarbital, mephobarbital, and metharbital: Biotransformation. In *Antiepileptic Drugs* (Ed.) Woodbury, D.M., Penry, J.K. & Schmidt, R.P. pp.311-317. New York: Raven Press.

Menkes, J.H. (1980) *Textbook of Child Neurology*. Philadelphia: Lea & Febiger. 695 pp.

Merlis, J.K. (1970) Proposal for an international classification of the epilepsies. *Epilepsia*, 11, 114-119.

Merlis, J.K. (1972) Treatment in relation to classification of the epilepsies. *Acta Neurologica Latinoamericana*, 18, 42-51.

Metrakos, K. & Metrakos, J.D. (1961) Genetics of convulsive disorders: II. Genetic and electroencephalographic studies in centrencephalic epilepsy. *Neurology*, 11, 474-483.

Montouris, G.D., Fenichel, G.M. & McLain, L.W.,Jr. (1979) The pregnant epileptic: A review and recommendations. *Archives of Neurology*, 36, 601-603.

Murphy, J.E., Bruni, J. & Stewart, R.B. (1981) Clinical utility of six methods of predicting phenytoin doses and plasma concentrations. *American Journal of Hospital Pharmacy*, 38, 348-354.

Nelson, K.B. & Ellenberg, J.H. (1976) Predictors of epilepsy in children who have experienced febrile seizures. *New England Journal of Medicine*, 295, 1029-1033.

Nelson, K.B. & Ellenberg, J.H (1981) The role of recurrences in determining outcome in children with febrile seizures. In *Febrile Seizures* (Ed.) Nelson, K.B. & Ellenberg, J.H. pp.19-25. New York: Raven Press.

Newmark, M.E. & Penry, J.K. (1980) Catamenial epilepsy: A review. *Epilepsia*, 21, 281-300.

Newmark, M.E. & Porter, R.J. (1982) Clinical research trends in the genetics of epilepsy. In *Genetic Basis of the Epilepsies* (Ed.) Anderson, V.E., Hauser, W.A., Penry, J.K. & Sing, C.F. pp.161-168. New York: Raven Press.

Newmark, M.E., Theodore, W., DeLaPaz, R., Sato, S., DiChiro, G., Brooks, R.A., Kessler, R.M. & Porter, R.J. (1982) Positron emission computed tomography (PECT) in refractory complex partial seizures. *Transactions of the American Neurological Association*, 106, 34-37.

Niedermeyer, E. (1976) Immediate transition from a petit mal absence into a grand mal seizure: Case report. *European Neurology*, 14, 11-16.

Nishimura, R.N., Ishak, K.G., Reddick, R., Porter, R., James, S. & Barranger, J.A. (1979) Lafora disease: Diagnosis by liver biopsy. *Annals of Neurology*, 8, 409-415.

Painter, M.J., Pippenger, C., Wasterlain, C., Barmada, M., Pitlick, W., Carter, G. & Abern, S. (1981) Phenobarbital and phenytoin in neonatal seizures: Metabolism and tissue distribution. *Neurology*, 31, 1107-1112.

Penry, J.K (1973) Behavioral correlates of generalized spike-wave discharge in the electro-encephalogram. In *Epilepsy: Its Phenomena In Man* (Ed.) Brazier, M.A.B. pp.171-188. New York: Academic Press.

Penry, J.K. & Dreifuss, F.E. (1969) Automatisms associated with the absence of petit mal epilepsy. *Archives of Neurology*, 21, 142-149.

Penry, J.K. & Porter, R.J. (1977) Intensive monitoring of patients with intractable seizures. In *Epilepsy: The Eighth International Symposium* (Ed.) Penry, J.K. pp.95-101. New York: Raven Press.

Penry, J.K. & Newmark, M.E. (1979) The use of antiepileptic drugs. *Annals of Internal Medicine*, 90, 207-218.

Penry, J.K. & Porter, R.J. (1979) Epilepsy: Mechanisms and therapy. *Medical Clinics of North America*, 63, 801-812.

Penry, J.K. & So, E.L. (1981) Refractoriness of absence seizures and phenobarbital. *Neurology*, 31, 158.

Penry, J.K., Porter, R.J. & Dreifuss, F.E. (1972) Ethosuximide: Relation of plasma levels to clinical control. In *Antiepileptic Drugs* (Ed.) Woodbury, D.M., Penry, J.K. & Schmidt R.P. pp.431-441. New York: Raven Press.

Penry, J.K., Porter, R.J. & Dreifuss, F.E. (1975) Simultaneous recording of absence seizures with video tape and electroencephalography: A study of 374 seizures in 48 patients. *Brain*, 98, 427-440.

Penry, J.K., Porter, R.J., Sato, S., Reddenbough, J. & Dreifuss, F.E. (1976) Effect of sodium valproate on generalised spike-wave paroxysms in the electroencephalogram. In *Clinical and Pharmacological Aspects of Sodium Valproate (Epilim) in the Treatment of Epilepsy* (Ed.) Legg, N.J. pp.158-164. MCS Consultants: Tunbridge Wells.

Pippenger, C.E., Penry, J.K., White, B.G., Daly, D.D. & Buddington, R. (1976) Interlaboratory variability in determination of plasma antiepileptic drug concentrations. *Archives of Neurology*, 33, 351-355.

Pippenger, C.E., Paris-Kutt, H., Penry, J.K. & Daly, D. (1977) Proficiency testing in determinations of antiepileptic drugs. *Journal of Analytical Toxicology*, 1, 118-122.

Pisciotta, A.V. (1982) Carbamazepine: Hematological toxicity. In *Antiepileptic Drugs*, Second edition (Ed.) Woodbury, D.M., Penry, J.K. & Pippenger, C.E. pp.533-541. New York: Raven Press.

Pond, D. (1981) Epidemiology of the psychiatric disorders of epilepsy. In *Epilepsy and Psychiatry* (Ed.) Reynolds, E.H. & Trimble, M.R. pp.27-32. Edinburgh: Churchill Livingstone.

Porro, M.G., Kupferberg, H.J., Porter, R.J., Theodore, W.H. & Newmark, M.E. (1982) Phenytoin: An inhibitor and inducer of primidone metabolism in an epileptic patient. *British Journal of Clinical Pharmacology*, 14, 294-297.

Porter, R.J. (1980a) Methodology of continuous monitoring with videotape recording and electroencephalography. In *Advances in Epileptology: The Xth Epilepsy International Symposium* (Ed.) Wada, J.A & Penry, J.K. pp.35-42. New York: Raven Press.

Porter, R.J. (1980b) Etiology and classification of epileptic seizures. In *Epilepsy Updated: Causes and Treatment* (Ed.) Robb, P. pp.1-10. Chicago: Year Book Medical Publishers.

Porter, R.J. (1981) Pharmacokinetic basis of intermittent and chronic anticonvulsant drug therapy in febrile seizures. In *Febrile Seizures* (Ed.) Nelson, K.B. & Ellenberg, J.H. pp.107-118. New York: Raven Press.

Porter, R.J. (1982) General Principles: Clinical efficacy and use of antiepileptic drugs. In *Antiepileptic Drugs* (Ed.) Woodbury, D.M., Penry, J.K. & Pippenger, C.E. pp.167-175. New York: Raven Press.

Porter, R.J. (1983a) Efficacy of antiepileptic drugs. In *Epilepsy* (Ed.) Ward, A.A.,Jr., Penry, J.K. & Purpura, D. pp.225-237. New York: Raven Press.

Porter, R.J. (1983b) Antiepileptic Drug Development Program. In *Orphan Drugs and Orphan Diseases: Clinical Realities and Public Policy* (Ed.) Brewer, G.J. pp. (in press). New York: Alan R. Liss.

Porter, R.J. (1983c) Intractable seizures. In *Epilepsy: Diagnosis and Management* (Ed.) Browne, T.R. & Feldman, R.G. pp. 355-361. Boston: Little, Brown.

Porter, R.J. & Layzer, R.B. (1975) Plasma albumin concentration and diphenylhydantoin binding in man. *Archives of Neurology*, 32, 298-303.

Porter, R.J. & Penry, J.K. (1977) Efficacy and choice of antiepileptic drugs. In *Advances in Epileptology, 1977: Psychology, Pharmacotherapy, and New Diagnostic Approaches* (Ed.) Meinardi, H. & Rowan, A.J. pp.220-231. Amsterdam: Swets & Zeitlinger.

Porter, R.J. & Penry, J.K. (1980) Phenobarbital: Biopharmacology. In *Advances in Neurology, Vol 27: Antiepileptic Drugs—Mechanisms of Action* (Ed.) Glaser, G.H., Penry, J.K. & Woodbury, D.M. pp.493-500. New York: Raven Press.

Porter, R.J. & Kupferberg, H.J. (1982) Other succinimides: Methsuximide and phensuximide. In *Antiepileptic Drugs*, Second Edition (Ed.) Woodbury, D.M., Penry, J.K. & Pippenger, C.E. pp.663-671. New York: Raven Press.

Porter, R.J. & Pitlick, W.H. (1982) Anticonvulsants. In *Basic & Clinical Pharmacology* (Ed.) Katzung, B.G. pp.239-254. Los Altos: Lange Medical Publications.

Porter, R.J. & Sato, S. (1982) Secondary generalization of epileptic seizures. In *Advances in Epileptology: XIIIth Epilepsy International Symposium* (Ed.) Akimoto, H., Kazamatsuri, H., Seino, M. & Ward, A.A.,Jr. pp.47-48. New York: Raven Press.

Porter, R.J. & Penry, J.K (1983) Petit mal status. In *Advances in Neurology, Vol 34: Status Epilepticus—Mechanisms of Brain Damage and Treatment* (Ed.) Delgado-Escueta, A.V., Wasterlain, C.G., Treiman, D.M. & Porter, R.J. pp.61-67. New York: Raven Press.

Porter, R.J., Wolf, A.A.,Jr. & Penry, J.K. (1971) Human electroencephalographic telemetry: A review of systems and their applications and a new receiving system. *American Journal of Electroencephalographic Technology*, 11, 145-159.

Porter, R.J., Penry, J.K. & Dreifuss, F.E. (1973) Responsiveness at the onset of spike-wave bursts. *Electroencephalography and Clinical Neurophysiology*, 34, 239-245.

Porter, R.J., Penry, J.K. & Wolf, A.A.,Jr. (1976) Simultaneous documentation of clinical and electroencephalographic manifestations of epileptic seizures. In *Quantitative Analytic Studies in Epilepsy* (Ed.) Kellaway, P. & Petersen, I. pp.253-268. New York: Raven Press.

Porter, R.J., Penry, J.K. & Lacy, J.R. (1977) Diagnostic and therapeutic reevaluation of patients with intractable epilepsy. *Neurology*, 27, 1006-1011.

Porter, R.J., Schulman, E.A. & Penry, J.K. (1980) Phenytoin monotherapy in intractable epilepsy. In *Advances in Epileptology: XIth Epilepsy International Symposium* (Ed.) Canger, R., Angeleri, F. & Penry, J.K. pp.419-422. New York: Raven Press.

Porter, R.J., Theodore, W.H. & Schulman, E.A. (1981) Intensive monitoring of intractable epilepsy: A two-year follow-up. In *Advances in Epileptology: XIIth Epilepsy International Symposium* (Ed.) Dam, M., Gram, L. & Penry, J.K. pp.265-268. New York: Raven Press.

Porter, R.J., Penry, J.K., Lacy, J.R., Newmark, M.E. & Kupferberg, H.J. (1979) Plasma concentrations of phensuximide, methsuximide, and their metabolites in relation to clinical efficacy. *Neurology*, 29, 1509-1513.

Post, R.M. & Cutler, N.R. (1979) Pharmacology of acute mania. *Clinical Pharmacology, Vol 4.* (Ed.) Klawans, H.L. pp.39-81. New York: Raven Press.

Raskin, N.H. & Fishman, R.A. (1976) Neurologic disorders in renal failure. *New England Journal of Medicine*, 294, 143-148.

Rasmussen, T. (1975) Surgical treatment of patients with complex partial seizures. In *Advances in Neurology, Vol 11: Complex Partial Seizures and Their Treatment* (Ed.) Penry, J.K. & Daly, D.D. pp.415-449. New York: Raven Press.

Reiser, S.J. (1978) Humanism and fact-finding in medicine. *New England Journal of Medicine*, 299, 950-953.

Reynolds, E.H. & Trimble, M.R. (1981) *Epilepsy and Psychiatry*. Edinburgh: Churchill Livingstone. 379 pp.

Riikonen, R. (1982) A long-term follow-up study of 214 children with the syndrome of infantile spasms. *Neuropediatrics*, 13, 14-23.

Riley, T.L. (1980) Lying About Epilepsy. (Letter to the editor.) *New England Journal of Medicine*, 303, 644.

Riley, T.L. (1982) Syncope and hyperventilation. In *Pseudoseizures* (Ed.) Riley, T.L. & Roy, A. pp.34-61. Baltimore: Williams & Wilkins.

Riley, T.L. & Roy, A. (1982) *Pseudoseizures*. Baltimore: Williams & Wilkins. 231 pp.

Riley, T.L., Porter, R.J., White, B.G. & Penry, J.K. (1981) The hospital experience and seizure control. *Neurology*, 31, 912-915.

Robins, M.M. (1962) Aplastic anemia secondary to anticonvulsants. *American Journal of Diseases of Children*, 104, 614-624.

Rodin, E.A. (1975) Psychosocial management of patients with complex partial seizures. In *Advances in Neurology, Vol 11: Complex Partial Seizures and Their Treatment* (Ed.) Penry, J.K & Daly, D.D. pp.383-414. New York: Raven Press.

Rodin, E.A., Rim, C.S. & Rennick, P.M. (1974) The effects of carbamazepine on patients with psychomotor epilepsy: Results of a double-blind study. *Epilepsia*, 15, 547-561.

Rose, A.L. & Lombroso, C.T. (1970) Neonatal seizure states: A study of clinical, pathological, and electroencephalographic features in 137 full-term babies with a long-term follow-up. *Pediatrics*, 45, 404-425.

Rowan, A.J., Binnie, C.D., de Beer-Pawlikowski, N.K.B., Goedhart, D.M., Gutter, T., van der Geest, P., Meinardi, H. & Meijer, J.W.A. (1979) Sodium valproate: Serial monitoring of EEG and serum levels. *Neurology*, 29, 1450-1459.

Saint-Hilare, J.M., Gilbert, M., Bouvier, G. & Barbeau, A. (1980) Epilepsy and aggression: Two cases with depth electrode studies. In *Epilepsy Updated: Causes and Treatment* (Ed.) Robb, P. pp.145-176. Chicago: Year Book Medical Publishers.

Sato, S., Dreifuss, F.E. & Penry, J.K. (1976a) Prognostic factors in absence seizures. *Neurology*, 26, 788-796.

Sato, S., Penry, J.K. & Dreifuss, F.E. (1976b) Electroencephalographic monitoring of generalized spike-wave paroxysms in the hospital and at home. In *Quantitative Analytic Studies in Epilepsy* (Ed.) Kellaway, P. & Petersen, I. pp.237-251. New York: Raven Press.

Sato, S., White, B.G., Penry, J.K., Dreifuss, F.E., Sackellares, J.C. & Kupferberg, H.J. (1982) Valproic acid versus ethosuximide in the treatment of absence seizures. *Neurology*, 32, 157-163.

Schmidt, D. (1981) The effect of pregnancy on the natural history of epilepsy: Review of the literature. *Epilepsia*, 22, 365.

Serrano, E.E. & Wilder B.J. (1974) Intramuscular administration of diphenylhydantoin: Histologic follow-up studies. *Archives of Neurology*, 31, 276-278.

Serrano, E.E., Roye, D.B., Hammer, R.H. & Wilder, B.J. (1973) Plasma diphenylhydantoin values after oral and intramuscular administration of diphenylhydantoin. 23, 311-317.

Sheehan, D.V. (1982) Current concepts in psychiatry: Panic attacks and phobias. *New England Journal of Medicine*, 307, 156-158.

Sheridan, P.H., Tsay, J. & Porter, R.J. (1983) Dose-dependent dystonic movements induced by carbamazepine. *Neurology*, 33 [Suppl 2]: 198.

Sherwin, A.L. (1982) Ethosuximide: Relation of plasma concentration to seizure control. In *Antiepileptic Drugs*, Second Edition (Ed.) Woodbury, D.M., Penry, J.K. & Pippenger, C.E. pp.637-645. New York: Raven Press.

Sherwin, A.L., Robb, J.P. & Lechter, M. (1973) Improved control of epilepsy by monitoring plasma ethosuximide. *Archives of Neurology*, 28, 178-181.

Simon, D. & Penry, J.K. (1975) Sodium di-N-propylacetate (DPA) in the treatment of epilepsy: A review. *Epilepsia*, 16, 549-573.

Suchy, F.J., Balistreri, W.F., Buchino, J.J., Sondheimer, J.M., Bates, S.R., Kearns, G.L., Stull, J.D. & Bove, K.E. (1979) Acute hepatic failure associated with the use of sodium valproate: Report of two fatal cases. *New England Journal of Medicine*, 300, 962-966.

Swanson, P.D., Luttrell, C.N. & Magladery, J.W. (1962) Myoclonus—A report of 67 cases and review of the literature. *Medicine*, 41, 339-356.

Taylor, J. editor (1931) *Selected Writings of John Hughlings Jackson, Vol 1: On Epilepsy and Epileptiform Convulsions*. London: Hodder and Stoughton. Reprint 1958. New York: Basic Books.

Teare, A.J. (1980) True gestational epilepsy: A case report. *South African Medical Journal*, 57, 546-547.

Terrence, C.F., Rao, G.R. & Perper, J.A. (1981) Neurogenic pulmonary edema in unexpected, unexplained death of epileptic patients. *Annals of Neurology*, 9, 458-464.

Theerman, M.R., Shuster, A. & Fanale, J.E. (1979) Nephrotoxic effects of computerized tomographic brain scan. (Letter to the editor.) *New England Journal of Medicine*, 300, 45-46.

Theodore, W.H. & Porter, R.J. (1983a) Removal of sedative-hypnotic antiepileptic drugs from the regimens of patients with intractable epilepsy. *Annals of Neurology*, 13, 320-324.

Theodore, W.H. & Porter, R.J. (1983b) Withdrawal of sedative-hypnotic antiepileptic drugs from outpatients. In *The Rational Prescription of Antiepileptic Drugs* (Ed.) Shorvon, S. & Birdwood, G. (In press). Berne: Hans Huber.

Theodore, W.H., Porter, R.J. & Penry, J.K. (1981) Complex partial seizures: A videotape analysis of 108 seizures in 25 patients. *Neurology*, 31, 108.

Theodore, W.H., Porter, R.J. & Penry, J.K. (1983a) Complex partial seizures: Clinical characteristics and differential diagnosis. *Neurology*, (in press).

Theodore, W.H., Schulman, E.A. & Porter, R.J. (1983b) Intractable seizures: Long-term follow-up after prolonged inpatient treatment in an epilepsy unit. *Epilepsia*, (in press).

Theodore, W.H., Newmark, M.E., Sato, S., Brooks, R., Patronas, N., DeLaPaz, R., DiChiro, G., Kessler, R.M., Margolin, R., Gratz, E. & Porter, R.J. (1983c) [18F]-Fluorodeoxyglucose positron emission computed tomography in refractory complex partial seizures. *Annals of Neurology*, (in press).

Toone, B. (1981) Psychoses of epilepsy. In *Epilepsy and Psychiatry* (Ed.) Reynolds, E.H. & Trimble M.R. pp.111-137. Edinburgh: Churchill Livingstone.

Treiman, D.M. & Delgado-Escueta, A.V. (1983) Complex partial status epilepticus. In *Advances in Neurology, Vol. 34: Status Epilepticus—Mechanisms of Brain Damage and Treatment* (Ed.) Delgado-Escueta, A.V., Wasterlain, C.G., Treiman, D.M. & Porter, R.J. pp.69-81. New York: Raven Press.

Trimble, M.R. (1981) *The Psychopathology of Epilepsy*. West Sussex: Geigy Pharmaceuticals. 278 pp.

Troupin, A.S. (1976) The choice of anticonvulsants—A logical approach to sequential changes. In *A Textbook of Epilepsy* (Ed.) Laidlaw, J. & Richens, A. pp.248-271. Edinburgh: Churchill Livingstone.

Troupin, A.S., Ojemann, L.M. & Dodrill, C.B. (1976) Mephenytoin: A reappraisal. *Epilepsia*, 17, 403-414.

Tower, D.B. (1978) Epilepsy: A world problem. In *Advances in Epileptology, 1977: Psychology, Pharmacotherapy, and New Diagnostic Approaches* (Ed.) Meinardi, H. & Rowan, A.J. pp.2-26. Amsterdam: Swets & Zeitlinger.

Turnbull, D.M., Rawlins, M.D., Weightman, D. & Chadwick, D.W. (1982) A comparison of phenytoin and valproate in previously untreated adult epileptic patients. *Journal of Neurology, Neurosurgery, and Psychiatry*, 45, 55-59.

Van Buren, J.M., Wood, J.H., Oakley, J. & Hambrecht, F. (1978) Preliminary evaluation of cerebellar stimulation by double-blind stimulation and biological criteria in the treatment of epilepsy. *Journal of Neurosurgery*, 48, 407-416.

Van Woert, M.H. & Rosenbaum, D. (1979) L-5-Hydroxytryptophan therapy in myoclonus. In *Advances in Neurology, Vol 26: Cerebral Hypoxia and Its Consequences* (Ed.) Fahn, S., Davis, J.N. & Rowland, L.P. pp.107-122. New York: Raven Press.

Vining, E.P.G., Mellits, E.D., Cataldo, M.F., Dorsen, M.M., Spielberg, S.P. & Freeman, J.M. (1982) Effects of phenobarbital and sodium valproate on neuropsychological function. *Abstracts of Joint Annual Meeting of the American Electroencephalographic Society and American Epilepsy Society, Phoenix, 1982*. p.50.

Volpe, J.J. (1981) *Neurology of the Newborn*. Philadelphia: W.B. Saunders. 648 pp.

Walton, J.N. (1977) *Brain's Diseases of the Nervous System*, Eighth Edition. New York: Oxford University Press. 1,277 pp.

Ward, A.A.,Jr. (1983) Perspectives for surgical therapy of epilepsy. In *Epilepsy* (Ed.) Ward, A.A.,Jr., Penry, J.K. & Purpura, D. pp.371-375. New York: Raven Press.

Weinberger, J. & Lusins, J. (1973) Simultaneous bilateral focal seizures without loss of consciousness. *Mt. Sinai Medical Journal*, 40, 693-696.

Wilder, B.J. & Ramsay, R.E. (1976) Oral and intramuscular phenytoin. *Clinical Pharmacology and Therapeutics*, 19, 360-364.

Wilder, B.J. & Buchanan, R.A. (1981) Methsuximide for refractory complex partial seizures. *Neurology*, 31, 741-744.

Wolf, M.W. (1981) Prevention of recurrent febrile seizures with continuous drug therapy: Efficacy and problems of phenobarbital or phenytoin therapy. In *Febrile Seizures* (Ed.) Nelson, K.B. & Ellenberg, J.H. pp.127-134. New York: Raven Press.

Woodbury, D.M. & Kemp, J.W. (1982) Sulfonamides and derivatives: Acetazolamide. In *Antiepileptic Drugs*, Second Edition (Ed.) Woodbury, D.M., Penry, J.K. & Pippenger, C.E. pp.771-789. New York: Raven Press.

Index